Vitamins

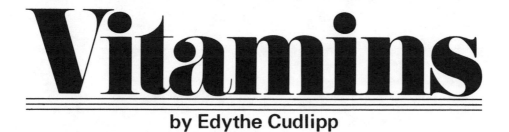

Vitamins

by Edythe Cudlipp

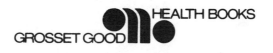

GROSSET GOOD HEALTH BOOKS

Publishers · GROSSET & DUNLAP · New York
A FILMWAYS COMPANY

CONTENTS

PART I   AN INTRODUCTION TO
            VITAMINS AND MINERALS   1
PART II   VITAMINS
   Vitamin A   13
   Vitamin B Complex   16
      Vitamin B_1 (Thiamine)   17
      Vitamin B_2 (Riboflavin)   19
      Vitamin B_3 (Niacin)   21
      Vitamin B_5 (Pantothenic Acid)   23
      Vitamin B_6 (Pyridoxine)   25
      Vitamin B_{12} 27
      Vitamin B_c (Folic Acid)   29
      Biotin   31
   Vitamin C   33
   Vitamin D   36
   Vitamin E   38
   Vitamin K   40

PART III MINERALS

Calcium   43
Chlorine   45
Chromium   47
Cobalt   48
Copper   49
Fluorine   50
Iodine   51
Iron   53
Magnesium   55
Manganese   57
Molybdenum   58
Phosphorus   59
Potassium   61
Selenium   63
Sodium   64
Sulfur   66
Zinc   67
Other Trace Elements   69
Glossary   71

Part I
An Introduction to Vitamins and Minerals

Vitamins and minerals are essential to the body's functions and to all-around good health. However, if we don't get enough of them, or if the body is unable to use what it gets, vitamin-deficiency diseases can result. But, vitamins and minerals are not a panacea for every human condition, disease, or contagion to which we are exposed.

For example, "tired blood" has been the slogan for peddling a wide variety of remedies. As a result, iron was one of the first food supplements to receive more than its share of attention because of its role in the formation of red blood cells or hemoglobin. The B vitamins were also touted for that reason during the 1940s and 1950s—and still are. Vitamins C and E have in the past been in the spotlight and have emerged again as popular vitamins.

In all cases, some justification may exist for a few of these claims, but there are many more claims that cannot be scientifically proven or justified. Iron is a good case of how a mineral supplement can be exploited.

For example, although both men and women need iron, women during their child-bearing years do need more iron than men, as certain advertisments claim. A man who eats a balanced diet generally gets the iron he needs from the foods he eats. The amount needed by a menstruating woman usually exceeds her iron intake in foods. So women probably do need supplemental iron, at least during their child-bearing years. But the phrase "tired blood" is an advertising gimmick. There is no such thing.

Red blood cells "live" 120 days, after which time the iron is absorbed by the bone marrow and is "reborn" in new blood cells. This is a constant process. And, since all red blood cells are not reproduced at the same time, blood cannot get tired. If you actually feel tired, you may be anemic—or you may not be getting enough rest. But it is *you* who is tired, not your blood.

Sorting fact from fiction where vitamins and minerals are concerned, therefore, can be difficult. To understand our needs for vitamins we must know about the vitamins and minerals, how many we need, how these recommendations are set, and by whom they are set. We also need to know what foods contain which vitamins and minerals and about preparing and cooking these foods to preserve their vitamin and mineral content insofar as is possible.

Specific information is given for individual vitamins and minerals in Parts II and III. But first there is some general information that we should know, beginning with the various stages of nutrition.

The first stage is related to our diet, the food that we take into our bodies. How good—or bad—that diet is accounts for whether we are well nourished or not, because nutrition is the result of the processes involved in the taking in and making use of foods. The first stage, then, is "ingestion."

The second stage is "digestion." In digestion, complex foods are broken down into simple nutrients or substances that the body can use: proteins must be broken down into amino acids; carbohydrates, into simple sugars such as glucose; and fats, into fatty acids and glycerol. Each type of food is broken down by specific "enzymes" or "catalysts" found in the digestive juices.

The third stage is "absorption." In this stage, the products of digestion—simple sugars, amino acids, and fatty acids—are absorbed through the intestinal walls into the bloodstream and are carried by the blood to those places in the body where they are needed, used, and/or stored.

The fourth stage is "metabolism." Metabolism includes all the processes involved in using substances entering the body, including the growth, repair, and maintenance of body tissues and bodily activities.

Vitamins and minerals are necessary to our diet because they are necessary to digestion, absorption, and metabolism. Thus, we need food to live, but we also need certain foods that are rich in vitamins and minerals to help us live healthy lives.

VITAMINS and MINERALS

Vitamins are organic compounds, which means they have a carbon origin and are composed of several elements (carbon, hydrogen, oxygen, and sometimes nitrogen). They are manufactured by plants and are found in both plant and animal products. Yet, although they are found in foods, they don't contribute calories any more than they add to the weight or change the taste of foods. Taking vitamin supplements, therefore, does not change our food requirements, because we still need the foods in which the vitamins are found to live; food is the source of energy, with vitamins helping to convert the food into energy, among other functions.

To begin with, proteins, fats, and carbohydrates must be broken down by enzymes into the substances the body uses. Certain vitamins act as coenzymes, which are substances that activate enzymes. Without the coenzymes, the enzymes cannot do their work.

That's only one function. In childhood, vitamins are vital to the growth and development of the body—including its bone structure, tissues, and nervous system. But we never outgrow our need for vitamins. All our lives they are responsible for the healthy maintenance of the body and for the healing of wounds and injuries. The circulatory system, both blood vessels and blood, needs vitamins, too. So do the endocrine glands, which produce many chemicals called hormones. For all of these reasons, the lack of vitamins can result in a variety of diseases and conditions. For every vitamin, in fact, there is a deficiency disease.

Minerals, fundamentally, are elements or substances that are unique and basic. Each element consists of one atom that cannot be broken down any further. Elements in their pure form, however, are rarely found. Some, in fact, such as chlorine, are poisonous. Yet the body needs chlorine. So, what the body uses is a mineral compound containing chlorine in a safe form—sodium chloride, or table salt. Salt is used by the body, therefore, to meet its needs of both sodium and chlorine.

Minerals, unlike vitamins, are found in soil and water. The mineral content of foods —whether protein, carbohydrate, or fat—depends on the soil in which fruits and vegetables are grown and on the feed which animals eat, in the case of meat and dairy products.

Minerals cannot be substituted for vitamins or vice versa, although their purposes in the body are somewhat similar. In some instances they may need each other to be effective. For example, vitamin D is necessary for the formation of healthy bones and teeth, but healthy bones and teeth also need calcium.

Many foods contain several vitamins and minerals, although some foods may be better sources of certain vitamins and minerals than others. Leafy green vegetables, for instance, contain almost all vitamins and quite a few essential minerals. So does milk. All foods contain sodium chloride, some much more than others.

A few vitamins and minerals, such as vitamin D and iodine, are less widespread in foods. Their scarcity is why foods may be fortified with them. They are also why a balanced diet is so important: the wider the variety of foods we eat, the better the chances are that we will get all the vitamins and minerals we need.

Vitamins and minerals, then, generally have much in common. They are found as nutrients in foods, and they are essential to the life processes of the body. There are also differences.

Vitamin Facts

In 1913, researchers found that rats fed a diet low in natural fats didn't grow normally and their eyes were inflamed. Supplementing the diet with butter fat or cod-liver oil relieved the eye condition. The particular constituent was isolated. Because it was necessary to life (*vita*, in Latin) and belonged to the amine family of chemicals, it was called vitamine, becoming known as vitamin A. New constituents were later discovered. New names were suggested, but the word vitamin, with the e dropped, stuck.

The next vitamin became B and so on, giving vitamins the designations with which we are now most familiar. Not all vitamins were designated alphabetically, however. Sometimes, they were named after their disease-prevention properties. Thus, the vitamin that prevented pellagra (a disease characterized by skin, gastrointestinal, neurologic, and mental symptoms) was called Pellagra-Preventive or P.P. Factor.

As more became known about vitamins, what had been thought to be single vitamins were found to be several vitamins. Vitamin A, for example, was found in two forms—*retinol* and *carotene*. In addition, some vitamins thought to be separate vitamins were found to belong to the same family. The largest family is the B-complex vitamins. Thus, the P.P. Factor began to be called vitamin B_3, when it was found to be similar in chemical structure to vitamins in that family.

Presently still another classification is becoming common—and that is to call vitamins after their chemical structure. As a result, the P.P. Factor, or vitamin B_3, is now better known as niacin.

Vitamins, therefore, may be listed alphabetically, such as vitamins A, B, C, D, E, and K, as has been done in this book. They may also be listed by their chemical names. In addition, they may be grouped together according to whether they are fat-soluble or water-soluble.

Fat-soluble vitamins are vitamins that dissolve only in fats and are not affected by water. They are absorbed by the small intestine, along with fats, and they are stored in the body's fatty tissues. Anything that interferes with the digestion and absorption of fats will interfere with the body's ability to use these vitamins. Because these vitamins can be stored, we don't have to eat foods containing them every day; our bodies have a reserve.

The fat-soluble vitamins are vitamins A, D, E, and K. We should know which ones they are for two good reasons. First, because they are stored in the body, a deficiency disease may take a long time to show up. Second, because they are stored, the body will go on storing them or trying to store them even when the body's saturation point is reached. The fact that they are not soluble in water means that they cannot be excreted with the body's wastes. The result is that an excess of these vitamins can be as hazardous as a deficiency. (See megavitamins and individual vitamins.)

Water-soluble vitamins are those vitamins that dissolve only in water. For this reason they can be—and are—excreted by the body in urine and perspiration. Thus, they are not stored in any quantity by the body. Once the body has reached the limit it can use, it simply eliminates the excess. At the same time, the body does seem to store some of the excess. (See megavitamins and individual vitamins.)

Water-solubility means more to us than the fact that our bodies tend to excrete the excess.

It also means that we should take care in preparing and cooking foods with these vitamins. The vitamins will dissolve out if vegetables are left to soak in water. They will also dissolve out in cooking. (See storage and preparation of foods.)

Vitamins are natural constituents of foods. And the assumption is that they are not made in the body. This assumption is generally true, although some vitamins are also manufactured by the body. Only one vitamin, vitamin D, however, is made in quantity, but it needs help. That help is provided by sunlight, which is a provitamin of vitamin D. (See vitamin D.) A provitamin is a substance that comes before, and is necessary to making, a vitamin. In the same sense, a vitamin can be a prohormone.

Mineral Facts

Minerals are also essential to our bodies and our health. All plant and animal life, from one-celled organisms to man, require minerals to live. Thus, certain quantities are necessary to health and nutrition—and too much, in some cases, can be as hazardous as too many of some vitamins.

The minerals that our bodies need include both what are called essential minerals and trace elements. Common to both minerals and trace elements is that they are found in soil and water as well as in the cells of plants and animals. The difference between them is the amount our bodies need. Our bodies require larger amounts of essential minerals than of trace elements. For this reason essential minerals are also called macronutrients, whereas trace elements are also called micronutrients.

Minerals compose four percent of our body weight. More than one-third, thirty-nine percent, is calcium.

VITAMIN AND MINERAL REQUIREMENTS— RECOMMENDED DAILY ALLOWANCES

After the first discovery of vitamins in this century, more and more of these constituents of foods were found. And more and more of

the age-old diseases that had plagued man began to be cured as a result.

The discovery of vitamin B (first isolated in 1936), especially niacin, led to the elimination of pellagra, which had been a virtual plague in the South.

The identification of thiamine, another B vitamin, brought about a cure for beriberi, a devastating disease that was common in the Orient.

Vitamin C was recognized as the specific constituent that prevented and cured scurvy, although fruits rich in vitamin C had unknowingly been used long before for their curative powers.

Among the minerals, iron and calcium were found to be important for blood and for bone development and growth.

At the same time, little was known about how much of any of these and other vitamins and minerals might be necessary for the maintenance of good health and for growth and development in children. Then, just before the United States entered World War II in 1941, concern about vitamin and mineral requirements grew. For one thing, the nutrition of the general population had to be protected in case of shortages. For another, the nutrients necessary for good health were important in planning and devising military rations.

This dual need resulted in the start of the National Nutrition Program. Under this program, the Food and Nutrition Board was established under the National Research Council of the National Academy of Science. The board was given authority to draw up recommended daily allowances (RDA), the RDA now found on vitamin labels and on labeling for a variety of foods, including cereals, milk, and yogurt.

The board published its first listing of the RDA in 1941, based on research current then. The vitamins included were vitamin A; thiamine, riboflavin, and niacin of the B vitamin family; and vitamin C. The minerals included were calcium and iron.

Since 1941, scientists and nutritionists have learned much more about these and other vitamins and minerals. As a result, the list of RDA has been updated several times, to include many more vitamins and minerals. In addition, as new research is scientifically proven, amounts have been changed. The process is a constant one; the RDA listings are given in Parts II and III here, and are based on the latest tables drawn up by the Food and Nutrition Board.

The RDA are based on several factors. First is a person's height and weight. The average adult male is considered to be 69 inches tall (5'9"), to weigh 147 to 154 pounds, and to eat about 2,700 calories a day. The average adult female is considered to be 65 inches tall (5'5"), to weigh 128 pounds, and to eat about 2,000 calories a day. The needs of both men and women decrease slightly after age 51.

Children's needs are also based on height and weight. Another factor, however, is based on their requirements at different ages.

Naturally, not everyone fits these averages. A larger man or woman who is very active will need more calories as well as more nutrients. A smaller man or woman who is sedentary will require less. For these reasons, the Food and Nutrition Board emphasizes that the daily allowances are only recommended.

The RDA also contain leeway in their recommendations. In some instances, they may be high. For example, the United Nations Food and Agricultural Organization (FAO) and the World Health Organization (WHO) have drawn up recommendations, especially for underdeveloped and developing countries, based on minimum necessary amounts. As a result, the Joint FAO-WHO Expert Group gives much lower requirements in general for both vitamins and minerals.

Both the Food and Nutrition Board and the FAO/WHO use the same measurements based on the metric system. Grams are used, rather than ounces, because much smaller amounts can be measured. For example:

1 ounce = 28.3 grams
1 gram (gm) = 1,000 milligrams (mg)
1 milligram = 1,000 micrograms (μg)

Since most recommendations are measured in milligrams and a few in micrograms, all allowances are relatively tiny. The fact that they may even be infinitesimal, however, does not change how essential they are or how powerful those infinitesimal amounts may be, which is why the RDA should be treated with respect.

An exception to these measurements is the measurement used for the fat-soluble vitamins A, D, and E. These are usually measured in international units (IU), a designation originally defined by a League of Nations committee that tried to establish guidelines for vitamins before World War II. One IU is roughly equivalent to one milligram. In addition, vitamin A nowadays is also measured in what are called retinol equivalents (RE). Retinol is the basic chemical compound of which vitamin A is composed, and RE are based on the metric system. (See Part II, vitamin A.)

Meeting the RDA

Because vitamins and minerals are found in foods, and in water in the case of minerals, we should technically be able to meet the RDA if we eat a balanced diet. A balanced diet means that each day the following foods should be eaten:

2 or more servings of: Meat, poultry, fish, eggs, dried beans or peas, or nuts.

4 or more servings of: Whole grain or enriched breads and cereals.

4 or more servings of: Fruits and vegetables that include a citrus fruit or other source of vitamin C, a dark green or deep yellow vegetable that contains vitamin A (every other day is enough for this because vitamin A is stored in the body), and other vegetables, including potatoes, and fruits.

In addition, a reasonable amount of fats, including vegetable oils, is necessary.

Some of these sources may be hidden. For example, cakes and sauces may contain milk, eggs, and fats and can be considered as having the requirements of a balanced diet.

Such a diet eaten daily means we should meet the RDA of vitamins and minerals. The only exception is for women during their child-bearing years who cannot get their RDA of iron out of foods. At the same time, there may be exceptions to the balanced diet:

1. Although meat, poultry, fish, eggs, dried beans or peas, or nuts can be substituted for one another, this does not mean a person can get all the needed vitamins on a purely vegetarian diet. Meat and dairy products are a major source of some vitamins, especially vitamin B$_{12}$; not eating them can result in a vitamin deficiency. (See Part II, vitamin B$_{12}$.)

2. Not all of us eat a balanced diet every day. For one reason or another, we may skip meals or overload on such foods as pizza that are rich in calories but not in vitamins and minerals. We also may have certain food prejudices and dislikes. Any of these reasons may make taking supplemental vitamins advisable.

3. Certain medically approved diets call for the avoidance of some foods. The balanced diet, although still considered nutritionally ideal, is relatively rich in fats, and high-fat diets have recently come under attack as contributing to heart disease, stroke, and hardening of the arteries. The "prudent diets," recommended by the American Heart Association and others, are based on avoiding animal fats and reducing the amount of foods that are rich in cholesterol. Cholesterol is actually a blood fat found in eggs, red meat, and organ meats, among other foods. Other diets may also be medically advisable. For example, persons with stomach or intestinal disorders may be advised by their physicians to avoid foods with roughage. Thus, again, supplementary vitamins and minerals may be necessary.

4. Even if we do eat a balanced diet, we still may not get the RDA of vitamins and minerals. One reason is the way foods are processed. Whole grains are rich in vitamins and minerals, but milling and bleaching the grains to make white flour destroys almost all of the vitamins and minerals because they're found in husks and coverings. This is why most white flours are enriched, to make sure we get the essential nutrients that are lost in processing. Enriched breads, then, are good vitamin and mineral sources, despite processing.

5. Other foods may lose vitamins and minerals for other reasons. To begin with, the fresher vegetables and fruits are, the more nutrients they contain. Even the few days necessary to send fresh fruits and vegetables from the fields

or orchards to stores will result in some loss of vitamins. Then, if they are stored longer at home, even more vitamins will be lost. Preparing them causes further loss of water-soluble vitamins.

6. Reliance on convenience foods can mean we are getting fewer vitamins than we think, too. Water-soluble vitamins, in particular, are lost easily in processing convenience foods.

Supplementary Vitamins and Minerals

A case can be made, therefore, for taking supplementary vitamins. Although the American diet is considered the best in the world, it still may lack some essential vitamins, even among economically well-off people, as some recent studies have found. Fast and convenience foods have lessened the nutritional value of what we eat. Even if we eat well, we can eat better.

That we don't eat as well as we might doesn't mean that vitamin-deficiency diseases are ravaging us. The vast majority of physicians in the United States actually have never seen a vitamin-deficiency disease.

The story is told, for example, of a physician who diagnosed a case of scurvy, the vitamin-C-deficiency disease, when he was interning in a major New York hospital. Physicians from all over the city came to see the patient because they had never seen a person with scurvy. Such diseases are rare, but what may be less rare than we think is subclinical or marginal deficiencies.

Subclinical or marginal deficiencies are difficult to diagnose. The person's only complaints may be of tiredness or general malaise: "I just don't feel well," is a typical complaint. There are no specific symptoms for a person to complain of—or for a physician to spot. The deficiency is borderline, not severe enough for the classic symptoms of the vitamin deficiency to appear. The complaints, in fact, may be so vague that they could be symptomatic of a dozen or more other conditions, giving the physician little to go on to look for a source of the complaints or in making a diagnosis.

Thus, again, there is some justification for taking supplementary multivitamins. Taking such supplements, however, means taking them carefully.

Megavitamins

Although taking vitamin supplements has a rationale, taking doses above and beyond—far beyond—the RDA does not. Large doses (or *megavitamins*, as amounts greatly above the RDA are called) can be too much of a good thing and can be harmful.

Over the years, megavitamins have gone through certain fads. Among the first vitamins to be used—and abused—were the B vitamins. As therapy, usually prescribed by psychiatrists, megavitamins have neither gained scientific approval nor proved clinically successful.

Vitamin B_{12} has been particularly abused. It is not a cure-all, but a specific cure. The only condition for which it is necessary is pernicious anemia, although it may also be used to treat chronic alcoholics who develop anemia because of an inadequate diet. Whatever the reason may be for a physician to prescribe vitamin B_{12}, self-dosing with large amounts of the vitamin is false therapy. Even so, it has gained popularity as a remedy for hangovers and is said to prevent fatigue, even though there is no medical proof that it helps either condition physically. It may help psychologically, but so would any remedy that a person believed in. There is also no proof that any other vitamin in massive doses prevents or cures hangovers or fatigue or any other condition or disease to which human beings are subject—except specific vitamin-deficiency diseases.

Yet, there is proof that some vitamins can be toxic or poisonous. The Food and Drug Administration's National Clearinghouse for Poison Control Centers receives some 4,000 reports of vitamin poisonings each year. About 3,200 of these cases involve children.

Some children may take the vitamins on their own, such as the little boy in Kansas who took a whole bottle of children's vitamins because he wanted to grow stronger, faster. Instead, he went to a hospital and spent two days in intensive care, recovering from vitamin A and iron poisoning.

Other children may take them under adult guidance. For example, the misguidance of a grandmother who owned a health-food store led to her four-year-old grandson being hospitalized, after months of illness before that, with vitamin A poisoning. The grandmother had let the child help himself generously to the natural vitamins in the store. There have also been cases of children and young people with symptoms of brain tumors who were later found to have vitamin A poisoning.

Then, why do people take megavitamins? Hangovers and fatigue aren't the only reason. Young people mistakenly take them as a cure for acne, which they are not. Older people take them to prevent "neuritis" or nervousness, osteoarthritis, osteoporosis, mental disorders, heart disease, and even impotence. The most common megavitamin usage today, however, is probably vitamin C to prevent or treat colds. None of these uses has been proven effective, and some overdosing may be harmful.

Just how harmful megavitamins can be depends partly on the vitamin involved. The oil-soluble vitamins, for example, should never be taken in amounts greater than the RDA, unless they are taken under a physician's supervision. Once the body has absorbed and stored the maximum it can handle, the excess still accumulates in tissues. Since fat-soluble vitamins are not soluble in water, they cannot be excreted in urine or perspiration.

What can happen with megadoses of vitamin D is a good example of what dangers exist from excess vitamins in the system. Vitamin D is necessary to help the body make use of calcium. It is, therefore, essential to healthy bones and teeth. It is also found in the blood, because calcium is absorbed from the intestines and is carried by the blood to where it is needed.

Too much calcium in the blood results in a condition called hypercalcemia, in which the soft tissues may calcify or harden. The kidneys, because they cannot excrete the vitamin D or calcium, may be seriously injured. These results don't happen at once, of course. In the meantime, the person may suffer from weakness, lethargy, loss of appetite, and constipation. These symptoms, moreover, may persist for months after the person has stopped taking vitamin D.

Vitamin A can be just as dangerous. Extended megadoses can cause dry and cracked skin, headaches, and bone pain. In children, it can retard growth instead of promoting it. In both children and adults, megadoses over a period of time can even increase pressure inside the skull, causing symptoms that mimic brain tumors ("pseudotumor cerebri").

Vitamin E, which is also oil-soluble, is being taken by some users in amounts ten times the RDA and sometimes in amounts even greater than that. The effect of such megadoses is not known, because vitamin E is still a greatly unexplored vitamin. What is known is that almost all of the many claims for it cannot and have not been proven in controlled scientific studies. In rats and other animals it does seem to be related to its effect on sterility and fertility conditions and to certain diseases, but these studies cannot be duplicated in humans. Thus, the scientific assumption is that it may work differently in animals and humans.

Some claims for vitamin E, furthermore, cannot be proven even in animals. In one instance, vitamin E has been touted as an antiaging vitamin. Yet rats fed vitamin E do not live longer and show no difference in how quickly or slowly they age than do rats who are not fed vitamin E. It also is not a "sex" vitamin, as has been claimed. As many researchers point out, psychology is a potent force in sexual performance. A person who strongly believes vitamin E—or carrots—may help, *may* be helped, although it may be less so because of the vitamin E than because of the mental state.

At the same time, vitamin E—long called the vitamin in search of a disease—does have a disease it is used to treat. That disease, however, affects only premature infants. (See Part II, vitamin E.)

Vitamin C, in megadoses of 500 to 4,000 milligrams, was heralded a few years ago as a cold preventive. If a person caught cold anyway, it was said to alleviate the symptoms.

The original evidence was anecdotal, based on the experiences of the Nobel Prize-winning chemist Linus Pauling and his wife. Since then, many studies have been performed. Despite using similar, double-blind experiments (in which one group takes vitamin C and another,

a placebo, or sugar pill, with neither knowing which one it was getting), no two experiments have come up with the same results. More reliable studies need to be done before anyone can say scientifically that vitamin C is an effective cold preventive and treatment.

The fact that vitamin C is water-soluble and we excrete excess amounts has led to the rationale that, if vitamin C doesn't help, it can't hurt. Nevertheless, long-term research has tended to show that this rationale may be untrue. Large doses over a long period of time may be harmful. Such overdoses may cause kidney stones. They may also make accurate testing for diabetes difficult, since vitamin C in the urine disguises or distorts the sugar levels. Large doses can also distort the result of a vital blood test to determine certain types of intestinal cancer and other stomach disorders. They may also have a long-range effect. (See Part II, vitamin C.) For these reasons, anyone taking megadoses of vitamin C (or any other vitamin, for that matter) should inform his or her physician of the fact, especially before undergoing tests.

Megavitamins, therefore, are no cure-all and can be dangerous. We should take any claims for them with healthy skepticism, keeping in mind the side effects and possible side effects of such large doses.

Remember, the body is a remarkable machine in which many systems coordinate with one another and depend on one another. It needs a balanced diet to function at its best—and that diet includes a balance of vitamins and minerals. Too much of any one element may be enough to throw the balance off and affect the functioning of the body.

Self-dosing with vitamins can be dangerous in another respect. Symptoms of vitamin deficiency are often similar to symptoms from other causes. Anemia is not the only reason for fatigue. Bleeding gums may be a symptom of vitamin C deficiency, but it also may be a sign of infection or disease. Lethargy and loss of appetite are common vitamin-deficiency symptoms, and they are also symptoms of a variety of other conditions, both physical and psychological. In fact, most subclinical or marginal vitamin-deficiency symptoms are general, but so can be symptoms due to other conditions. Thus, taking large doses of vitamins won't necessarily help—and selfdosing could be like playing with fire, not only because large amounts may be harmful, but they may keep a person from seeking medical help.

In short, anyone is mistaken who thinks that if a little of a vitamin is a good thing, a lot will do much more. Megavitamins are to be avoided, unless there is a distinct medical reason for taking them, such as taking vitamin B$_{12}$ for pernicious anemia. A multivitamin supplement is generally safe, whereas megavitamins are far different and may be hazardous if used incorrectly.

Natural or Organic Vs. Synthetic Vitamins

If megavitamins are controversial, so are natural, or organic, vitamins. All vitamins are organic compounds, which means they have a carbon origin. Once the organic structure is known, the various elements can be combined in the laboratory to synthesize the original compound. They are still organic compounds, though.

The term *organic* as used by natural or organic vitamin manufacturers is misleading in that it has nothing to do with vitamins being organic compounds. It is used to designate vitamins derived from natural sources and sources grown without the use of chemical fertilizers and pesticides. Thus, natural or organic vitamins come from such sources as wheat germ and wheat-germ oil, which are rich in a variety of vitamins.

Organic, therefore, is a misleading term because both synthetic and natural vitamins are organic compounds. The confusion has led to a clarification by the National Nutritional Foods Association, a trade association of health-food retailers, distributors, and manufacturers. It prefers the term *organically grown* to "organic," with organically grown to mean as follows:

"Organically grown food produced on humus-rich soil whose fertility has been maintained with organic materials and natural mineral fertilizers. No pesticides, artificial fertilizer, or synthetic additives shall be used in the production of organic food."

As to which is best—natural or synthetic vitamins—we must first ask: Is there a difference between them? Almost all scientists, nutritionists, and researchers in the field feel that there is no difference. Organic compounds *are* organic compounds, and our bodies don't know the difference. Those in favor of natural or organic foods claim the body makes better use of natural products. They feel synthetic vitamins are chemicals, to whose use they are opposed. One big difference between them, however—and it can be a very big one—is price.

Synthetic vitamins are inexpensively mass-produced under scientific controls for quality and strength. Natural or organic vitamins are much more expensive. If your body doesn't know the difference, your pocketbook certainly will.

· Another difference is quality control. Natural or organic vitamins may not always be produced under the best of conditions. In addition, what are you getting? The fact is the vitamins may not always be what the label claims and may contain synthetic vitamins.

The important factor in choosing either kind of vitamin is the label—reading it to make sure the bottle contains the RDA and no less or no more. That means checking the international units, milligrams, or micrograms that measure the biologic activity of the vitamin. In Part II, the RDA is given, along with the different names that the vitamins are called, for each specific vitamin.

Synthetic vitamins, especially those put out by large pharmaceutical companies, are usually well marked. Not all natural or organic vitamins are so clearly marked, as some natural vitamin manufacturers admit. For this reason, the National Nutritional Foods Association offers the following guidelines as to what is to be considered naturally derived (primarily from food) and synthetic (primarily from chemicals) sources of vitamins and minerals:

A. Vitamin A derived from fish liver, shark, or carotene oils is to be considered as naturally derived; all other sources to be considered synthetic.

B. Unfortified B vitamins derived solely from yeast, rice bran, and liver are to be considered as naturally derived; all other B vitamins except vitamin B_{12} (cobalamin) are to be considered synthetic. (Author's Note: Cyanocobalamin is the name for the original chemical structure of the compound. It has now been shortened to cobalamin.)

C. Vitamin C derived from glucose fermentation, including acerola, rose hips, or other plant sources is to be considered as naturally derived; however, the "Vitamin C" on any label must be dominant above any other food sources.

D. Vitamin D derived from fish liver oils, or an irradiation of yeast or vegetable oils is to be considered as naturally derived.

E. Vitamin E labeled as Mixed Tocopherols, D'Alpha Tocopheryl Acetate, or D'Alpha Tocopheryl Succinate from vegetable oils is to be considered as naturally derived. (Author's Note: All vitamin E is highly processed to separate the vitamin E from the vegetable or wheat-germ oil sludge. The result is that the chemical name is used. Furthermore, not all natural vitamin manufacturers would agree that all of the above forms are natural. At least one company insists that only the vitamin E marked as a form of D'Alpha tocopheryl is natural, with mixed tocopherols being synthetic.)

F. All minerals are to be considered as naturally derived; however, those containing sulphates are not recommended.

In short, anyone who wants natural vitamins has to look for far more than the RDA. The label has to be interpreted correctly because the term *natural* is not enough to tell what is inside the bottle. Another factor is how the vitamins are stored. If no preservatives are used, the vitamins could go rancid or spoil—even on the store shelf before you buy them. Synthetic vitamins, however, have a long shelf life and do not need special care in storage.

Cooking and Preparation of Foods

Although we may take vitamin supplements for a variety of reasons, we should not take them as a replacement for food. A balanced diet is still the best source of both vitamins and minerals.

Minerals in foods generally tend to be stable; that is, they are not lost, regardless of how the food is prepared and cooked. Any exceptions are noted under the specific minerals in Part III.

Vitamins are another matter. As a general rule, fat-soluble vitamins are more stable than water-soluble vitamins. Although any special precautions are noted under the specific vitamins, some factors hold true for almost all vitamins. These factors are important because they may mean we are not always getting all the vitamins that we could or we think we are. They can also influence the way we prepare our shopping lists and plan our menus.

Fresh foods contain the most vitamins, especially fruits and vegetables. The fresher they are, the more vitamins they have, because vitamins tend to be lost during storage. Apples stored for two or three months, for example, will retain only about one-third of their original amount of vitamin C. Storing apples, potatoes, carrots, cabbage, and other fruits and vegetables that can be put away in a cool place will help them retain more vitamins than storing them at room temperature.

How we prepare food also determines how many vitamins we are getting. The method of preparation doesn't drastically change the food's protein, carbohydrate, or fat content, but it can change the vitamin content.

An example is potatoes, which are a rich source of vitamin C. The way potatoes are cooked won't affect their calorie content; as long as they are prepared without sauces, baking or boiling makes no difference, as far as calories are concerned. It does, when it comes to their vitamin C.

First of all, the longer the potatoes are stored—the older the potatoes—the less vitamin C they will have. That loss cannot be prevented to a large extent. Other losses can be prevented. Potatoes that are scrubbed and baked in their skins retain the maximum vitamin C. Scrubbed and boiled potatoes, provided they are boiled quickly and in as little water as possible, are next best. Remember, vitamin C is water-soluble and is lost in water. Leaving the skins on potatoes in cooking helps them retain more vitamin C because the skins prevent it from dissolving out in the water.

Peeling potatoes before cooking will result in a greater loss of vitamin C. In addition, letting the peeled potatoes soak in cold water before cooking causes vitamin C to soak out, and cooking them in a lot of water and for a long time further slashes the vitamin C content of the potatoes when eaten.

The same cautions hold true for all cooked vegetables containing water-soluble vitamins. See the individual vitamins for specific suggestions.

As preferable as fresh fruits and vegetables may be from a nutrition standpoint, we all sometimes use prepared foods. Prepared foods vary widely in the amount of vitamins they retain, depending on the method.

Dehydrated foods retain the most vitamins, with freeze-dried foods keeping more vitamins than hot-air dried foods.

Frozen foods are next best. The major loss in freezing, however, occurs when foods are thawed.

Canned foods have the fewest vitamins, because vitamins are lost both in blanching foods before canning and in the canning process, which requires high heat. Reheating them causes a further loss, as it also does with fresh vegetables.

Peas are a good example. If fresh peas are cooked quickly, and in as little water as possible, the cooked peas will retain forty-four percent of their original vitamin C. If frozen peas are served, the peas retain seventeen percent when eaten: twenty-five percent is lost in blanching the peas before freezing, with another nineteen percent lost during freezing and thirty-nine percent lost in thawing and cooking. If canned peas are served, the peas retain six percent of their vitamin C; all the rest is lost in blanching, sterilizing and reheating, and in the liquid in which the peas are canned that is usually drained before serving.

So, if we serve and eat canned vegetables instead of fresh, and eat frozen foods (including TV dinners) instead of preparing from scratch, we are depriving ourselves of essential vitamins. Supplementing these foods with fresh salads and raw vegetables and fresh fruit will help.

Once all of these factors are taken into consideration—processing, preparation, and cooking—there is little difference in the loss caused by the method of cooking. Whether foods are cooked on top of the stove, in the oven, or even in a microwave oven, the vitamin content remains the same.

A few simple precautions, therefore, can help save as many vitamins as possible.

1. Use fresh fruits and vegetables, as fresh as possible and as often as possible.

2. Avoid letting fresh vegetables stand in water, either while awaiting cooking or to "crisp" them.

3. Cook vegetables in as little water as possible and as quickly as possible. Don't overcook them. If possible, save the water—to avoid throwing out the valuable nutrients in the cooking water—for soups, stews, and gravies.

4. Serve cooked foods as soon as possible.

5. Avoid reheating foods. Reheating causes even more vitamins to be lost in the second heating. This means preparing only what will be eaten in one meal. Leftover vegetables, however, can always be eaten cold or in salads.

Vitamin Antagonists or Antivitamins

Sometimes vitamins are lost for reasons that have nothing to do with storage, preparation and processing, and cooking. One of these reasons is that certain food substances "antagonize" the vitamins; that is, the substances act so that they make the vitamins unavailable to the body. One example is *avidin*, a substance found in raw (not cooked) egg whites. Avidin inhibits the action of *biotin*, a B-complex vitamin sometimes called vitamin H, in the body. For this reason, it is called a vitamin antagonist, or antivitamin. Cooking the egg white however, destroys the avidin.

Another reason that vitamins may not be able to do their work is the taking of certain antibiotics. The antibiotics not only kill the infectious bacteria but also attack the bacteria in the digestive track that are necessary to digest food properly and manufacture certain vitamins. The latter bacteria are not permanently affected, and the effect normally stops after the antibiotic is no longer being taken.

Vitamin antagonists may sometimes be used for medical reasons. Vitamin K is necessary for blood to clot. In certain types of heart disease and stroke, however, the clotting can be dangerous, adding to the possibility of a heart attack or stroke. In these cases, anticlotting or coagulant therapy may be necessary. If it is, the medication prescribed may be a vitamin antagonist or antivitamin of vitamin K.

All of this information is basic to understanding vitamins and minerals. It is, nevertheless, general information. Now for the specifics. Part II explains the vitamins, including the RDA, the foods in which they're found, and any other facts we should know. Part III does the same for minerals, both essential minerals and trace elements.

Part II
Vitamins

Vitamin A

WHAT IS VITAMIN A?

Vitamin A is actually several related compounds. Although it is found in both animal products and plants, natural or preformed vitamin A is found only in animal products. The form occurring in plants—both fruits and vegetables—is carotene, so called because it was first isolated from carrots. Carotene, which accounts for the yellow color in fruits and vegetables, such as oranges as well as carrots, is a provitamin or vitamin A precursor that is converted into vitamin A in the body during the digestive process.

Vitamin A is fat-soluble.

Why You Need Vitamin A

Vitamin A is essential to the development and healthy maintenance of the following.

Eyes and vision   The retina, the inner coat of the eye, contains light sensors or rods that control your ability to see in dim light or darkness. The rods manufacture visual purple, a pigment composed of protein and a substance manufactured by the body from vitamin A. Visual purple is bleached by light, decreasing night vision—the ability to see in the dark. In a unique chemical process, however, the rods restore visual purple with the help of vitamin A, enabling eyes to see in both light and darkness.

Epithelial tissue   Epithelial tissue forms the outer surface (epidermis) of the body and the linings of the body cavities and tubes and passageways. It has been called the body's first line of defense against disease. Since the cells of these tissues are constantly replacing themselves, a ready supply of vitamin A is necessary to help the cells reproduce healthy tissue. Each kind of epithelial tissue (such as skin, mucous membranes, cornea, digestive system,) has its own vitamin A requirements.

Bones and growth   Vitamin A is also necessary for the growth and development of bones. It helps manufacture the bone cells, called osteoblasts, which are essential to growth.

Recommended Daily Allowance
Average adult male   5,000 IU.
Average adult female   4,000-5,000 IU, with needs increasing to 5,000 IU during pregnancy and to 6,000-6,700 IU while nursing.
Children   Children require proportionately less, ranging from 1,400-3,500 IU, depending on age and size. They should never be given supplemental vitamin A in excess of the adult requirement without a physician's approval.

Effects of Vitamin A Deficiency

Eyes and vision   The first signs of a vitamin A deficiency occur in the eyes, and the eyes are the best symptom of the deficiency since other signs could be from other causes. A decreased ability to see in dim light and in bright light (such as the glare of the sun on snow) and night blindness are among the first signs of deficiency. The conjunctiva, the mucous membranes forming the socket of the eye, may also become dry.

If the deficiency continues untreated, the eyes will be further damaged by xerophthalmia, a disease in which the conjunctiva dries and the cornea starts to harden. In the later stages, the cornea softens and other parts of the eye (iris and lens) may be affected. If the deficiency is not treated, the cornea can be scarred permanently and blindness can occur.

Tissues   The skin may become dry, hard, and rough or scaly, especially on the arms and thighs. The inner linings of the body—the mucous membranes—may start to degenerate, resulting in increased susceptibility to infections, such as frequent colds. Remember, these membranes are the first line of defense against disease and infection.

Growth   Vitamin A deficiency in children results in a failure to grow.

Treatment   Vitamin A is prescribed at levels adequate to correct the deficiency. This treatment can only be prescribed by a physician who can monitor the levels of vitamin A, since too much vitamin A can be dangerous.

Effects of Excess Vitamin A

Since vitamin A is fat-soluble and is stored in the body, excess vitamin A is not excreted. Instead, it may accumulate in parts of the body that use vitamin A but do not have the capability of storing it. Amounts of vitamin A above 6,700 international units (8,000 IU for pregnant and nursing women), therefore, should be taken only under the supervision of a physician.

Too much vitamin A can result in a loss of appetite; hair loss; itchy, dry skin; increased fragility of the bones; pain in the bones and joints; and discoloring of the skin. Massive doses of vitamin A over a period of time can even cause symptoms similar to those of brain tumors, which would necessitate costly, delicate operations to rectify the condition. Other serious effects include enlargement of the liver and spleen. In women, the menstrual cycle can be disturbed. Ironically, in children, vitamin A, which is necessary for growth, can actually retard growth if taken in massive doses.

Too much of the provitamin carotene is usually not dangerous. Massive amounts, however, can cause the skin to turn yellow.

The effects of hypervitaminosis due to vitamin A usually disappear gradually when vitamin A is withheld from the diet.

Sources of Vitamin A

An average serving of the following foods contains more than the RDA of vitamin A: beef or calves' liver, raw or cooked carrots, boiled sweet potato, spinach or turnip greens.

Other foods rich in vitamin A are all yellow and dark green vegetables, yellow fruits (especially apples and cantaloupe), egg yolk, butter, cheese, and fish oils. Cod-liver and halibut oil are also rich in natural vitamin A and are often used as vitamin A supplements.

Cooking Precautions

Although foods containing vitamin A, including carotene, are sensitive to oxygen and air, acids, and high heat, they generally retain the vitamin in preparation and cooking. Nevertheless, vegetables should be cooked quickly and in as little water as possible to prevent loss of vitamin A.

History of Vitamin A

Vitamin A was the first fat-soluble vitamin recognized. In 1913, researchers noticed that rats on a diet lacking in natural fats failed to grow and their eyes became inflamed and infected. Adding butter fat or cod-liver oil to their diet corrected the effects. The factor responsible was named vitamin A. Until it was synthesized in the mid-1940s, fish oil was the primary source of supplemental vitamin A.

Other Facts

Retinol is the most common form of vitamin A as it occurs naturally and preformed in foods. Vitamin A may be measured in retinol equivalents instead of international units so that 1 RE = 3.33 IU.

Vitamin B Complex

The earliest documented evidence of a vitamin-deficiency disease, dating back to 2600 B.C. in China, is of beriberi. Today we know that the deficiency was due to vitamin B, and that vitamin B is not one vitamin but a complex of as many as twelve factors—and perhaps even more. Some of these factors are called vitamin B, such as vitamin B_1, vitamin B_2, and so on. Others are known by both numerical designations and chemical names, while still others are called primarily by chemical names.

The vitamin-B-complex family has certain properties in common. All B vitamins are:

1. Water-soluble.
2. Found in liver and yeast, both of which are rich sources, with dry yeast being the richest source.
3. Coenzymes or act as coenzymes. Enzymes, which are organic catalysts manufactured in the body, induce changes in other cells.

Coenzymes are selective and specific. For example, certain enzymes during the digestive process convert carbohydrates to glucose, the form of carbohydrates that fuels the body (such as the working of the brain) and provides energy for physical work. Other enzymes convert fats and proteins to forms the body can use. Coenzymes are compounds that activate specific or selective enzymes. Without the coenzyme, the particular process for which the enzyme is responsible cannot take place. Both enzymes and coenzymes are vital to the body's metabolism—the sum of the processes by which the body makes use of food, including the conversion of foods into products that the body can use or excrete.

The B-complex vitamins, each of which is considered separately in this section, are:

B_1 or thiamine
B_2 or riboflavin
B_3 or niacin
B_5 or pantothenic acid
B_6 or pyridoxine
B_{12} or cyanocobalamin or cobalamin
B_c or folacin or folic acid
Biotin (sometimes called vitamin H)
Or other organic compounds sometimes considered to be, or included in, the family of B vitamins.

Vitamin B₁ (Thiamine)

WHAT IS VITAMIN B₁ OR THIAMINE?

Vitamin B$_1$, or thiamine, as it is more commonly called, is a coenzyme essential to the converting of carbohydrates (sugars and starches) into energy and fuel. It is the member of the B-vitamin family responsible for preventing beriberi, a dysfunctioning of the nervous system. It is found in a wide range of animal and plant products, although rarely in abundance. In plant products, it is found in the bran covering that is removed in processing white flour and in polishing rice to make it white, which is why these products and foods containing them are enriched to replace the thiamine.

Thiamine is water-soluble. It is not stored in the body in appreciable quantities.

Why You Need Thiamine

Thiamine is essential to the proper functioning of the nervous system and the heart. It is absorbed through the small intestine and is present in the blood, liver, kidneys, heart, and brain, which store minute quantities that are rapidly depleted. Because thiamine in excess of the body's daily needs is excreted, you must include foods containing thiamine in your daily diet.

Recommended Daily Allowance

Average adult male	1.4-1.5 mg, with the needs decreasing slightly after the age of 51.
Average adult female	1.0-1.1 mg, with the needs increasing by 0.3-0.5 mg daily during pregnancy and while nursing. As with men, needs decrease slightly after 51 years.
Children	Infants require 0.3 mg daily, with needs increasing through childhood to adult RDA at age 11.

Effects of Thiamine Deficiency

Thiamine deficiency may be the most common of all vitamin deficiencies because it is processed out in the milling of wheat and other grains. The early symptoms include depression, irritability, loss of appetite, fatigue, constipation, and tenderness of muscles. The accumulation of certain acids in the brain, for whose disposal thiamine is essential as a coenzyme, can lead to marked disability of the nervous, circulatory, and digestive systems. The memory can also be affected. Such symptoms vanish quickly with the supplementation of thiamine to the diet.

If a thiamine deficiency goes untreated, beriberi is the result. This deficiency disease is rarely seen in Western countries, thanks to thiamine supplements in food, especially bread and flour. Because thiamine is so essential to general metabolism, all of the body's systems are involved in beriberi. There may be neuritis, nerve lesions, paralysis, digestive difficulties, heart problems, and fatigue. Again, thiamine can help the symptoms to disappear.

Effects of Excess Thiamine

Because thiamine is water-soluble, excess thiamine is excreted, mainly through the urine. The skin may also excrete some thiamine through perspiration.

Thiamine injections may cause adverse reactions. For this reason, it is rarely given intravenously.

Sources of Thiamine

The richest sources are dry yeast and wheat germ. Other good sources are the outer layers of seeds as well as nuts, legumes, most vegetables (especially potatoes), and some meats. The meats that supply the most thiamine include pork, liver, and organ meats. Enriched breads and cereals are also good sources.

Cooking Precautions

Care should be taken in preparing foods so that thiamine is not lost in preparation, such as in removing the outer layer of seeds and legumes. Heat also destroys thiamine. For example, the loss of thiamine in the crust of bread can be thirty percent, compared to a seven percent loss in the rest of the bread. Meats lose thiamine under heat, and milk loses it during pasteurization.

Thiamine is particularly sensitive to alkalis. Thus, in cooking vegetables, baking soda should never be used. It may keep vegetables brightly colored and attractive, but it destroys the food value. However, the bright and natural color of vegetables can be retained if they are not overcooked.

History of Thiamine

During the nineteenth century, physicians in different countries began to relate certain foods to beriberi. In the 1880s, a Japanese marine medical officer associated the large number of beriberi cases and deaths from it to diet. He helped reorganize the diet on a special training ship, decreasing the amount of rice and increasing the amount of vegetables, meat, and condensed milk. The only people sick on the ship's return, 287 days later, were those who refused the meat and milk. In the 1890s, a Dutch physician in Indonesia noticed chickens fed table scraps of polished rice suffered symptoms similar to people with beriberi. When they were fed brown rice scraps, however, they recovered. The case against polished rice was further established by an American physician in the Philippines in 1910. He fed bran extract to babies suffering from beriberi and cured them.

Thiamine was finally isolated and was first synthesized in 1936. It is now commonly used to enrich grain products.

Other Facts

Fruit is a poor source of thiamine and especially dried fruits, which are treated with sulfur that destroys thiamine.

Vitamin B$_2$ (Riboflavin)

WHAT IS VITAMIN B$_2$?

Vitamin B$_2$ is more generally known as riboflavin. It contains, and is part of, several enzymes that are associated with a wide variety of chemical reactions involved in the general metabolism of fats, carbohydrates, and proteins. A small amount of vitamin B$_2$ is manufactured in the digestive tract, although not enough to meet the body's requirements.

Riboflavin is water-soluble. Excess riboflavin is excreted. At the same time, small amounts are stored in the liver, spleen, kidneys, and cardiac muscle. This storage of riboflavin is maintained even when there is a vitamin deficiency, unlike thiamine, which is rapidly depleted.

Why You Need Riboflavin

Because riboflavin is involved in such a variety of metabolic processes, it is associated with the healthy maintenance of a number of tissues, including the skin. It is also essential to the health of the eyes and helps prevent light sensitivity.

Recommended Daily Allowance
Average adult male   1.6 mg
Average adult female   1.2 mg, with needs during pregnancy increasing to 1.5-1.7 mg.
Children   Needs increase from 0.4 mg in infancy to 1.8 mg in the teens, decreasing to adult dosage at age 22.
Note: Needs decrease slightly after age 51.

Effects of Riboflavin Deficiency

The eyes are most likely to show the first symptoms of riboflavin deficiency. The earliest symptoms are conjunctivitis, increased tearing, light sensitivity, burning and itching, eye strain and fatigue, and headaches. A common complaint is a feeling of "grittiness" under the lids. Notice that these symptoms are similar to those associated with vitamin A deficiency. This similarity illustrates one of the dangers of self-dosing with more vitamins than the RDA. Only a physician can determine the deficiency and prescribe the correct vitamin and dosage to correct it.

Other symptoms include paleness of the lips and mucous membranes of the mouth, along with splitting at the corners of the mouth and lip sores. Sores or lesions may also occur along the creases running from the nose to the mouth. Other tissues can be affected, too, such as around the eyes, on the ears, and on the genitals.

Symptoms disappear slowly with treatment by riboflavin, often supplemented with other B vitamins. Riboflavin deficiency, in fact, is usually not isolated but occurs along with a deficiency of other B vitamins.

Effects of Excess Riboflavin

Because riboflavin occurs in such small amounts in such a wide variety of animal and plant products, excess riboflavin is not a problem.

Sources of Riboflavin

The only food containing more than the RDA is liver. The next best source is milk. Since riboflavin is sensitive to light, however, you should buy milk in cartons or dark, not clear, bottles. In addition to organ meats and milk, good sources of riboflavin come from meats, cheese, leafy green vegetables, poultry, eggs, and fish. Flour, cereal, and bread have been enriched to provide another good source.

Cooking Precautions

Riboflavin is relatively stable during ordinary preparation and cooking. Vegetables should never be left standing in water or be cooked with a lot of water, to prevent as much loss as possible in the cooking water. Storing foods in dark areas will also prevent loss of riboflavin, because of its light sensitivity. Since alkaline solutions will drastically reduce the riboflavin contents of foods, avoid cooking with baking soda.

History of Riboflavin

Riboflavin was discovered to be a different vitamin from vitamin B_1 because of riboflavin's stability when heated: heat destroyed the factor preventing beriberi, but other growth factors (including riboflavin) remained. It was identified and synthesized in the 1930s.

Other Facts

Riboflavin, or vitamin B_2, is sometimes called vitamin G and lactoflavin, the latter because of its being found in milk.

Vitamin B₃ (Niacin)

WHAT IS VITAMIN B₃?

Vitamin B₃ is always called niacin. It is a part of the coenzymes that are essential to the metabolism of fats, carbohydrates, and proteins. Niacin can be made in the body from an amino acid called *tryptophan*, which is produced during the digestion of animal and vegetable protein. Tryptophan, therefore, is a provitamin, or precursor of niacin.

Niacin is water-soluble. Unlike thiamine and riboflavin, niacin is not stored at all in the body. Very little is excreted, however, because the body is extremely efficient in its use of niacin.

Why You Need Niacin

Many of the body's tissues require niacin, but it is primarily important for maintaining healthy skin and the functioning of the gastrointestinal tract and nervous system.

Recommended Daily Allowance

Average adult male   16-20 mg, depending on calorie intake and how active the man is.

Average adult female   12-14 mg, based on the same considerations, with needs during pregnancy and during nursing increasing by 2-4 mg.

Children   Infants require 5 mg, with their needs increasing with age to the adult level.

Effects of Niacin Deficiency

The result of severe niacin deficiency is pellagra, a disease characterized by dermatitis and gastrointestinal and neurological symptoms. Niacin deficiency, not so severe as to cause pellagra, has similar symptoms, with symptoms increasing in severity along with the deficiency.

The name *pellagra* means "rough skin" in Italian (the disease was first documented in Italy), but dermatitis is only one symptom. The mouth and tongue become inflamed; the stomach suffers upsets; and the skin will break out in dermatitis, with the dermatitis affecting both sides of the body, usually arms, legs, neck, and rib areas. Along with the physical symptoms are nervous symptoms, including insomnia and irritability. In advanced niacin deficiency, the nervous system becomes more involved and can result in insanity and death. The four *D*s of pellagra, are dermatitis, diarrhea, dementia, and death. Enriched flour, cereals, and bread have made this disease all but unknown in this country.

Effects of Excess Niacin

Although niacin is water-soluble, with the excess excreted, megadoses may be dangerous. It has been used experimentally to lower cholesterol and fat levels in the blood and to help prevent heart attacks in which these fats are a factor, because of its fat metabolism properties. Extremely high doses, however, seem to affect the heart muscle and could cause the very effect they are attempting to prevent. Large doses of niacin, in at least one reported incident, were associated with liver failure.

One form of niacin used as a vitamin supplement may cause hot flashes, but these are temporary.

Sources of Niacin

Meat, poultry, and fish are the best sources of niacin. Except for mushrooms and legumes, fruits and vegetables are not good sources. Milk and eggs, which do not contain much niacin, are rich in tryptophan, which the body converts into niacin. Enriched bread, cereals, and flour are also good sources.

Cooking Precautions

Niacin is a very stable vitamin, losing hardly any of its properties due to heat, light, alkalis, and even radiation. It is stable in cooking with baking soda. The biggest loss comes in cooking in water, since niacin dissolves in water.

History of Niacin

Although pellagra, the niacin-deficiency disease, was recorded as a disease as early as the eighteenth century, the relationship with niacin wasn't recognized until the 1920s. At that time patients and volunteers in whom pellagra had been induced were treated with dry yeast. Dry yeast cured the pellagra, but the curative factor in the yeast—niacin—was not isolated until 1937. Pellagra was once second only to rickets as a deficiency disease.

Other Facts

Niacin is sometimes called the Pellagra-Preventive, or P.P. factor. It was originally called *nicotinic acid* and still is referred to by that name at times. Because of the association of nicotinic acid with nicotine in tobacco (although nicotinic acid has no relationship to nicotine), niacin ("ni" from *nicotinic*, "ac" from *acid*, and "in" from *vitamin*) is now the much more common name.

In general, niacin is one of the most stable, easily obtainable, and cheapest vitamins, although it can be found in foods in a form that the body cannot use. Corn is one example. Thus, areas where corn is a staple often have high rates of pellagra cases. The exception is Mexico where corn is treated with lime water before tortillas, the basic food, are made. The lime water frees the niacin, thus enabling the body to make use of it.

In India, niacin deficiency is due to millet, which is a dietary staple there. Millet contains a large amount of an amino acid called *leucine*. Leucine increases the body's niacin needs, with a corresponding increase of niacin deficiency. So leucine, in this sense, is a niacin antagonist.

Vitamin B$_5$
(Pantothenic Acid)

WHAT IS VITAMIN B$_5$?

Vitamin B$_5$ is more commonly called *pantothenic acid*. The word *pantothenic* means "widespread," and this vitamin is part of a coenzyme found in a wide variety of food.

Pantothenic acid is water-soluble.

Why You Need Pantothenic Acid

Since pantothenic acid is basic and essential to metabolism and the body's use of fats, protein, and carbohydrates, it has a role in maintaining healthy skin, growth, and the development of the nervous system. It has also been associated with the red color of the blood's hemoglobin and with the formation of other acids and certain hormones needed by the body.

Recommended Daily Allowance

Required daily allowances of pantothenic acid have not been established. Anywhere from 5 to 10 milligrams are thought to be sufficient for healthy adults on the basis of the fact that up to 5 to 6 milligrams are excreted daily. Since the average diet is considered to contain 10 to 20 milligrams daily, most of us probably get enough if we eat a balanced diet.

Effects of Pantothenic Acid Deficiency

Although this deficiency has been induced in animals on a pantothenic-acid-deficient diet—causing hair loss and graying, intestinal ulcers, and damage to internal organs—these deficiencies have *not* been found in humans also on a pantothenic-acid-deficient diet. Deficiency in humans, in fact, is far less well documented. Symptoms only occur after about twelve weeks on a pantothenic-acid-deficient diet. They include fatigue, headaches, muscle cramps, gastrointestinal problems, and difficulties in coordination.

From the point of view of a specific deficiency disease that reacts solely to pantothenic acid, the only one noted as yet was in prisoners of war in the Far

East. The prisoners complained of "burning feet," and this symptom responded only to treatment with pantothenic acid and not to other B vitamins.

Effects of Excess Pantothenic Acid

Because the RDA has not been established, effects of excess pantothenic acid are also not known. Since it is water-soluble, however, the excess is excreted.

Sources of Pantothenic Acid

Most foods contain some pantothenic acid, although fruits are poor sources. The richest sources, as with most other B vitamins, are yeast, liver and organ meats (kidney and heart), and eggs, and salmon. Broccoli, pork, beef tongue, mushrooms, potatoes (white and sweet), peas, and peanuts are good sources, too. Wheat, rye, and soybean flour are excellent sources as well, depending on the milling, which can cause as much as half the pantothenic acid to be lost.

Cooking Precautions

Meats lose as much as one-third of their pantothenic acid during cooking. The pantothenic acid in vegetables is relatively stable, however, with little lost during preparation and cooking. It is not stable when used in combinations with acids and alkalis.

History of Pantothenic Acid

Pantothenic acid deficiency was first noticed as a dermatitis in chickens in the early 1930s. The dermatitis was cured by yeast, thus aligning the deficiency with the B vitamins. The exact factor responsible—pantothenic acid— was recognized in the late 1930s and was synthesized in 1940.

Other Facts

Pantothenic acid is sometimes called vitamin B_3 as well as vitamin B_5. Recently, it has been associated with stress and has been called the "antistress" factor. Even though this relationship has not been sufficiently backed up by scientific research, both synthetic and natural vitamin supplements that are called stress or antistress vitamins include it as a factor in B-complex vitamins.

Vitamin B₆ (Pyridoxine)

WHAT IS VITAMIN B_6?

Vitamin B_6 is also known as pyridoxine. It is actually three different coenzymes, one of which is necessary to convert tryptophan into niacin in the body. Another is essential in preventing anemia.

Pyridoxine is water-soluble.

Why You Need Pyridoxine

You need pyridoxine for the growth of red blood cells in the prevention of anemia. You also need pyridoxine for healthy teeth and gums and a healthy nervous system.

Recommended Daily Allowance

The amount of pyridoxine required is related to the amount of protein eaten. The average adult, however, requires 2 milligrams. During pregnancy and while nursing, women require 2.5 milligrams. Women on steroid birth-control pills may also have higher needs.

Because both human and cow's milk contain a low percentage of pyridoxine to protein, pediatricians may supplement infant diets with pyridoxine until the infants start on solid foods. Commercial formulas usually contain pyridoxine for this reason.

Effects of Pyridoxine Deficiency

Most diets contain adequate pyridoxine, with the result that pyridoxine deficiency is rarely seen. There are exceptions, though. Infants fed a formula with insufficient pyridoxine have been noticed to be nervous and irritable, with a tendency toward convulsions. These symptoms cleared up with supplemental pyridoxine.

In adults, deficiency symptoms include soreness of the mouth, dizziness, nausea, and weight loss. Nervous disturbances are also sometimes seen.

The only symptom noticed in women on birth-control pills is fatigue, which seems to make a higher intake advisable. Other drugs may affect the efficiency of the body in making use of pyridoxine as well, but these are relatively rare. In addition, some people have recently been found to have an "inborn error of metabolism" that interferes with their ability to make use of pyridoxine. All of these factors have resulted in much research now being done on the pyridoxine group.

Effects of Excess Pyridoxine

Although it is known that pyridoxine is excreted, very little is known about how it is absorbed. What, if any, the effects are of excess pyridoxine is a matter for more research to discover.

Sources of Pyridoxine

The best sources are pork, liver and organ meats, legumes, seeds, grains, potatoes, and bananas.

The major loss of pyridoxine in cooking happens during preparation when it is washed out. It is relatively stable at normal cooking temperatures, although there is more loss in roasted meats than in other kinds of prepared foods. It is not affected by light or oxygen, but alkalis (baking soda) and ultraviolet light will cause a loss. Foods also lose pyridoxine during the canning process. Pyridoxine is lost, too, in the sterilization (not pasteurization) of milk.

History of Pyridoxine

As already noted much research is needed, and is being done, on pyridoxine. It was first recognized as being part of the B-vitamin family and named vitamin B_6 in 1934. Pyridoxine was synthesized in the late 1930s.

Other Facts

The chemical names for two factors of vitamin B_6, other than pyridoxine, are pyridoxal and pyridoxamine. These names alone, or in combination, may be used in listings of vitamin contents of foods or vitamin supplements.

Inducing vitamin deficiencies in volunteers is the major method of determining what the deficiencies are. In some cases, the diet may be deficient. In other cases, the effects of the deficiency may be speeded up through the use of antagonists that block the effect of the vitamin. One reason that more research is needed is that pyridoxine-deficiency symptoms following the use of a deficient diet and those caused by antagonists are not the same. At this time, the only recognized symptoms of the deficiency are those already noted.

Vitamin B$_{12}$

WHAT IS VITAMIN B$_{12}$?

Vitamin B$_{12}$ is a coenzyme and contains cobalt, a natural trace element, leading to the name of cobamides being given to it and associated compounds. This cobalt makes vitamin B$_{12}$ unique. It is the only vitamin to contain an element other than carbon, hydrogen, oxygen, and sometimes nitrogen. It is one of the most powerful substances necessary to the metabolism of the body, with its RDA measured in micrograms instead of milligrams. To put it another way, 1 ounce equals 28.3 grams, or 28,300,000 micrograms—enough vitamin B$_{12}$ to provide the average adult RDA of 3 micrograms for almost 9 ½ million people. Chemically, it is also one of the most complicated of the water-soluble vitamins.

Vitamin B$_{12}$ is water-soluble. Despite its water-solubility, the vitamin can be stored in the liver.

Why You Need Vitamin B$_{12}$

Vitamin B$_{12}$ is essential to the formation of red blood cells in the bone marrow. It is also essential to the functioning of all cells and growth in children because of its role in making nucleic acid, an acid that is found in all cells and is responsible for the synthesis of the cells' RNA (ribonucleic acid) and DNA (deoxyribunucleic acid). RNA and DNA form the chemical basis of heredity and carry the cells' genetic information. Certain types of anemia are the result of defective DNA, owing to vitamin B$_{12}$ deficiency.

Vitamin B$_{12}$, in addition, is needed for the functioning of the nervous system and intestines.

Recommended Daily Allowance
Average adult male   3μg
Average adult female   3μg with needs increasing to 4μg during pregnancy and while nursing.
Children   0.3μg, in infancy, with needs increasing to adult RDA by early teens.

Effects of Vitamin B₁₂ Deficiency

Vitamin B_{12} deficiency leads to pernicious anemia and other forms of anemia. The most common symptoms are pallor of the skin, mucous membranes, and fingernails. Weakness, fatigue, dizziness, and headaches are also symptoms. In women, there may be a stopping of the menstrual cycle (amenorrhea). Anemia and the symptoms are cleared up with injections of vitamin B_{12}.

Another proof of the potency of the vitamin can be shown by the fact that the injections may contain as little as 6 micrograms vitamin B_{12}. In comparison, 20,000 to 50,000 micrograms of folic acid (see vitamin B_c), which is used to treat certain other types of anemia, is needed to be effective.

Effects of Excess Vitamin B₁₂

There are no known effects.

Sources of Vitamin B₁₂

Vitamin B_{12} is found only in meats and other animal products. Lean meat, liver, kidneys, milk, eggs, dairy products, salt-water fish, and oysters are rich sources of the vitamin.

Fruits and vegetables contain no vitamin B_{12}, although some of their products may be enriched with it. One danger of a strictly vegetarian diet (often called vegans) is that it can lead to a vitamin B_{12} deficiency. The lack of the vitamin in children is particularly dangerous. Nutritionists recommend that strict vegetarians include fortified soy milk in their diets or take vitamin B_{12} supplements. Lactovegetarian diets (containing milk, cheese, and other dairy products) and ovolactovegetarian diets (containing dairy products and eggs) generally contain enough vitamin B_{12}.

Cooking Precautions

The major loss of vitamin B_{12}, which is relatively stable, occurs when foods are soaked in water or marinated, allowing the vitamin to dissolve in the liquid.

History of Vitamin B₁₂

Liver was first used to treat anemia in 1926, leading to the theory that liver contained a special factor. This factor, vitamin B_{12}, was finally isolated in 1948.

Other Facts

Vitamin B_{12} is also called cobalamin and cyanocobalamin because of its chemical structure.

Vitamin B_{12} was the first vitamin purported to cure everything from a hangover to fatigue. As a result, it was also one of the first vitamins for which megatherapy (both in pills and by injection) became popular. Experts now recognize, however, that the average person gets adequate vitamin B_{12} through a normal balanced diet. Large doses, moreover, do not prevent or cure a hangover and won't relieve fatigue. Such doses may have a psychological effect, but the only time larger doses than the RDA will actually help is when the person is anemic. Anemia can only be diagnosed by a physician who can then prescribe the proper medication. In some cases of anemia, the preferred treatment may not be vitamin B_{12} at all, but folic acid.

Vitamin B$_C$ (Folic Acid)

WHAT IS VITAMIN B$_C$?

Vitamin B$_c$ is usually called folic acid. It is necessary to the manufacture of certain compounds found in RNA and DNA and for the complete use of certain amino acids by the body.

Folic acid is water-soluble. Limited quantities are stored in the liver.

Why You Need Folic Acid

You need folic acid for normal metabolism and to help manufacture red blood cells. It also aids in maintaining the proper functioning of the intestinal tract.

Recommended Daily Allowance

Average adult male   400 μg

Average adult female   400 μg, with needs increasing to 800 μg during pregnancy and to 600 μg while nursing.

Children   Infants require 50 μg, with needs increasing during childhood to the adult RDA at about age 10.

Effects of Folic Acid Deficiency

Certain types of anemia are associated with a folic acid deficiency. A less severe deficiency is sometimes found in elderly patients because of a poor diet. Sprue, a tropical disease of the intestines, is also caused by a folic acid deficiency. General symptoms, aside from anemia, are gastrointestinal disorders (diarrhea), and glossitis or inflammation of the tongue.

Effects of Excess Folic Acid

Excess folic acid is simply excreted.

Sources of Folic Acid

The richest sources are yeast, liver, kidneys, navy beans, and green leafy vegetables. Other good sources are nuts, fresh oranges, whole wheat products, milk, and eggs.

Cooking Precautions

Folic acid can be destroyed by heat, acids, and light. Since the folic acid in milk is destroyed in processing dried milk, children should not be given dried milk unless prescribed by a physician. Otherwise, folic acid is relatively stable in cooking, although some factors in folic acid can be destroyed in cooking and storage.

History of Folic Acid

Over the years, various factors related to the prevention of anemia have been noted. The first was found in 1935 and was called vitamin M. A year later, two others were found. One was called lactobacillus casei, and the other, folic acid. In the mid-1940s, all three were discovered to be the same factor and synthesized, with the name folic acid given to this. The B_c comes from the fact that it's found in liver and yeast.

Other Facts

In addition to the names above, folic acid is sometimes called folacin as well as PGA, the initials coming from the name for the pure form: pteroylglutamic acid.

Biotin

WHAT IS BIOTIN?

Biotin is a coenzyme essential to metabolism and especially to fat metabolism.

Biotin is water-soluble. Excretion can be greater than intake, indicating that it is probably manufactured inside the body.

Why You Need Biotin

The major purpose of biotin is in the metabolism of fats, carbohydrates, and proteins. Rich sources are milk, liver, kidney, leafy green vegetables, and egg yolks. Biotin deficiency is very rare, with the symptoms including mild skin disorders, some anemias, lassitude, depression, sleeplessness, and muscle pain.

Although not much is known about biotin, it is known that a substance called avidin, found in raw egg white, neutralizes biotin. For this reason, avidin is known as a biotin antagonist or antivitamin. Biotin deficiency, in fact, is found *only* when large amounts of *raw* egg whites are consumed. Avidin is destroyed by cooking, which means eating cooked egg whites will not cause a deficiency.

Required Daily Allowance

The average balanced diet contains up to 3,000 micrograms of biotin, which is considered adequate because it is also synthesized in the intestines. For this reason, an RDA of only 0.3 milligrams for adults is regarded as necessary. The RDA for young children is 0.15 milligrams.

Other Facts

Biotin is sometimes called vitamin H. Because it is found in yeast and liver, however, it is considered a member of the B-vitamin family.

OTHER B VITAMINS

Para-aminobenzoic acid (PABA) is sometimes listed as an individual B vitamin. Since research has found it's one of the forms of folic acid, it is no longer considered a separate vitamin by scientists and nutritionists. It is apt to be listed separately in listings of natural or organic vitamins.

The other actual members of the B-vitamin family are inositol, choline, and betaine. None has ever been associated with a vitamin-deficiency disease, and all are manufactured within the body. For these reasons, no RDA has been established for them.

Vitamin C

WHAT IS VITAMIN C?

Vitamin C is also called by its chemical name of ascorbic acid. It is used by a wide variety of tissues, each requiring different and specific amounts of vitamin C. Particularly high amounts of vitamin C are found in the tissues of such hormone-producing glands as the adrenal and pituitary glands and the pancreas, with the brain, kidneys, and spleen also having high amounts. Vitamin C acts as a preservative when added to certain foods.

Vitamin C is water-soluble. Once the tissues have reached their saturation level, the excess vitamin C is excreted in the urine and through perspiration. The fact that amounts above what the body can use are excreted doesn't mean that vitamin C in large amounts is harmless.

Why You Need Vitamin C

Vitamin C is essential to a wide range of life processes. To begin with, it prevents scurvy, a disease characterized by bleeding gums, loss of teeth, bleeding under the skin, bone fragility, and delayed healing of wounds and bones. Vitamin C is also necessary for the following:

1. The formation of collagen. Collagen is the "cement" or "glue" that holds cells and tissues together. It is needed for growth and for tissue repair. In the healing of wounds, tissues surrounding the wound will show an increase in vitamin C. A lack of vitamin C, therefore, slows healing. Collagen is also essential for healthy blood vessels.

2. Vitamin C breaks down iron into a form that the body can use.

3. It breaks down folic acid into folinic acid, the chemical compound that is used by the body. Vitamin C may also be necessary to the storage of this acid in the body.

4. It activates the metabolism of certain amino acids, which are found in protein and are necessary to the body in its manufacture of protein—skin and bones.

Recommended Daily Allowance

Average adult male   45 mg

Average adult female   45 mg, with needs increasing to 60 mg during pregnancy, and to 80 mg while nursing.

Children   Infants need 35 mg, increasing to 40 mg at 1 year and to adult RDA at 11 years.

Effects of Vitamin C Deficiency

Bleeding and sore gums and a sore mouth are the earliest signs. Other symptoms include lassitude, weakness, bleeding due to weakened walls of blood vessels, and irritability. Slowness of healing is also a symptom.

Effects of Excess Vitamin C

Although excess vitamin C is excreted, megadoses may have lingering effects. Bowel cancer, certain intestinal disorders, and adverse drug effects are detected by a common standard test of the presence of blood in the feces or stool. The results of this test, which is normally so reliable and is so simple that it is used about forty million times a year around the world, have been found to be questionable when the person is taking megadoses of vitamin C. Vitamin C makes the test turn out negative instead of positive, which could lead to a delay in medical treatment and even cost lives. For this reason, anyone undergoing a thorough medical examination or tests should not take vitamin C for forty-eight to seventy-two hours before testing and should inform the physician of the amount of vitamin C being taken. Large doses may also obscure routine tests, such as for sugar in the urine, which may indicate diabetes. For this reason, excess amounts of vitamin C could be dangerous for diabetics. Vitamin C has also been connected to the formation of kidney stones.

More recent studies of vitamin C in Canada have shown that megadoses may affect the DNA of cells, thus resulting in birth defects. Other studies indicate that with high doses, the excess vitamin C may possibly act as an antivitamin or antagonist of vitamin A, preventing vitamin A from performing its functions.

Sources of Vitamin C

The most commonly used fruits and vegetables are rich sources of vitamin C. An average serving of broccoli, fresh or frozen orange juice, strawberries, or turnip greens contains more than the RDA. Other excellent sources are other citrus fruits, currants, cantaloupe, leafy green vegetables (cabbage, lettuce, kale, collards, mustard greens), sweet peppers, and potatoes. Rose hips, usually found in natural- and health-food stores, are a rich source, too. The highest source is acerola or West Indian cherries, a fruit often neglected in its own environment.

Cooking Precautions

Vitamin C is one of the least stable vitamins. It is lost under heat, oxidation, drying, and storage. As a result, the amounts of vitamin C in foods vary, depending on how long they have been stored, how they have been stored, how they are prepared, and how they are cooked. The slightest alkalinity will destroy it. Peeling potatoes before cooking results in a major loss of vitamin C, as does slicing them. To prevent as much loss as possible, store fruits and vegetables containing vitamin C in a cool place and don't reheat them.

History of Vitamin C

Descriptions of diseases resembling scurvy occur in the Old Testament; Egyptian writings; in the pre-Christian writings of the Roman, Pliny; and in accounts of the Crusades. During the sixteenth and seventeenth centuries, scurvy was often confused with venereal disease and was even blamed on sailors bringing it back to Europe from abroad. Although scurvy is not contagious, its association with sailors had a certain accuracy. Sailors on long voyages did suffer more from scurvy than land dwellers. A British physician, Dr. James Lind, who was physician to the British fleet in the 1750s, first suggested the use of limes to prevent scurvy in 1753. Limes finally became optional additions to the diet of British sailors in 1795 and mandatory in 1884. The use of limes had another effect—that of British sailors being called "Limeys."

The discovery or use of a food supplement to

prevent scurvy, however, dates back further than Lind. American Indians used an infusion of steeped spruce or pine needles to prevent it at least four centuries ago. Also, European physicians before Lind had noted the effect of a decoction of pine needles and of citrus fruit. The substance was named vitamin C in 1920 and ascorbic acid in 1933 after it was synthesized.

Other Facts

The use of megadoses of vitamin C to prevent or alleviate the symptoms of colds was first advocated by Nobel Prize-winning chemist Linus Pauling. Investigations about its worth have been inconclusive. In some cases, investigators have found that people given large amounts of vitamin C have fewer colds, and those who do get colds have fewer uncomfortable symptoms. In other cases, vitamin C has had no effect. In short, a solid case cannot be made for or against the taking of large doses of vitamin C to prevent colds. The recent findings about vitamin C masking a vital blood test and its possible effects on DNA should be borne in mind, however. Also, few authorities—such as the American Medical Association, nutritionists, and others, including the Food and Nutrition Board of the National Academy of Sciences—recommend taking megadoses of any vitamin.

Increased amounts of vitamin C, nevertheless, may be indicated at times, although not in the megadose amounts sometimes advocated. For instance, vitamin C's role in healthy teeth and gums is well documented. Additional vitamin C may be beneficial before and after tooth extraction, to promote healing of gums, and before and after gum surgery. It may also be beneficial before and after surgery, since it is essential to the formation of the collagen required for healing broken bones and wounds. Vitamin C may also have a role in infectious diseases and in other infections, since controlled studies have shown that the body's level of vitamin C is low at these times. For example, in tuberculosis, the more advanced the disease, the more noticeable is the vitamin C deficiency. Thus, there is much more to be learned about the role of vitamin C.

Taking more than the RDA of vitamin C should be discussed with a physician. For one thing, persons with ulcers or intestinal disorders may be sensitive to vitamin C.

One further note: Although gum damage is a result of a vitamin C deficiency, extra vitamin C will neither prevent or "cure" periodontal disease. As already stated, most Americans consume more than enough vitamin C in their diet because it is one of the most commonly found vitamins in food.

Vitamin D

WHAT IS VITAMIN D?

Preformed vitamin D is found in relatively few foods. Unlike most vitamins, it is made in the body, with sunlight acting as a provitamin or precursor. Hence, it is sometimes called the "sunshine vitamin."

Vitamin D is oil-soluble. It is stored in the liver. Vitamin D is absorbed from the intestines, as are all fat-soluble vitamins, and requires bile salts for its absorption.

Why You Need Vitamin D

Vitamin D is necessary for the absorption of calcium and phosphorus by the bones, teeth, and blood. In children it helps maintain proper growth and is essential for the eruption of teeth. Vitamin D is also related to the prevention of dental cavities.

Recommended Daily Allowance

Infants, children, and young adults up to the age of twenty-three years have an RDA of 400 international units daily. In older children and adolescents, however, the vitamin-D-deficiency disease of rickets is almost unknown, but vitamin D is vital for infants and young children.

After the age of twenty-two, when adults have reached their maximum growth, supplementary vitamin D is not necessary and no RDA has been established. Vitamin supplements contain vitamin D on the basis that it should be taken in areas where there is little sunlight, in amounts up to 400 international units.

Women, during pregnancy and while nursing, should take supplemental vitamin D. The usual RDA at this time is 400 international units.

Elderly people, especially those who are sedentary, may need supplemental vitamin D. Its deficiency has been linked to osteoporosis, a disease of the elderly in which bones become fragile and break easily and the spine can become deformed.

Effects of Vitamin D Deficiency

Rickets, a disease that affects the ends of growing bones in infants and children, results from a vitamin D deficiency. Although the first overt symptoms are excessive sweating and gastrointestinal disturbances, the bones are actually affected earlier. The malformation of the bones results in a bowlegged condition. Soft bones, poor teeth, and other skeletal deformities may also be due to vitamin D deficiency.

Deficiency in elderly people has been linked to osteoporosis, as already noted.

Effects of Excess Vitamin D

Because vitamin D is fat-soluble and is stored in the body, excess vitamin D can be dangerous, leading to symptoms similar to those it prevents. Excess vitamin D can retard physical growth and can lead to mental retardation as well. Its first symptoms are generally nausea, weakness, stiffness, constipation, and hypertension or high blood pressure. Infants and children, therefore, should never take more than 400 international units daily, unless it is prescribed by a physician. The danger of excess should be weighed against needs.

Sources of Vitamin D

Since vitamin D is made in the body, with the help of the ultraviolet light in sunshine, sunlight is a source of vitamin D. Ultraviolet light rays may be filtered out of sunlight by fog, smoke, and even window glass. Natural skin pigments, know as melanin, which protect the skin of dark-skinned people in the tropics and are necessary for tanning in fair people, can also prevent absorption of ultraviolet rays. Thus, the darker the skin of a person living in the temperate zone, the greater may be the need for supplemental vitamin D in infants to prevent rickets.

Vitamin D is not widely distributed in foods, with vegetables, cream, butter, eggs, salmon, sardines, tuna fish, and liver containing only small amounts. For this reason, certain foods are fortified by irradiation with vitamin D, especially milk and some margarine. Fish-liver oil is the only rich source of vitamin D found naturally.

Cooking Precautions

Vitamin D is very stable during the cooking, storing, and aging of food. Warming vitamin-D-enriched milk for infants does not affect the vitamin. In addition, it is not affected by alkalis. Although ultraviolet irradiation is the primary means of fortifying foods with vitamin D, excess irradiation such as leaving fortified foods in sunlight is able to destroy the vitamin activity.

History of Vitamin D

Rickets has been recognized for centuries, as is shown by the number of Renaissance paintings depicting children with the typical bowlegged condition of rickets. The Dutch, in the early nineteenth century, used cod-liver oil as a preventive, and its use was later accepted by French and German physicians. Because physicians could not explain how and why cod-liver oil worked, it later fell into disfavor. Extensive research on vitamin D, including the effects of ultraviolet rays, was begun in the 1920s, leading to the vitamin's discovery in the 1930s.

Other Facts

Pure vitamin D is also called calciferol, the chemical name given to the compound. About ten different compounds actually have been found to be vitamin D active. The two most important compounds are ergocalciferol and cholecalciferol.

Vitamin E

WHAT IS VITAMIN E?

Vitamin E was known for years as "the vitamin without a disease." Later research found it to be an alcohol, known as tocopherol. The most active form is alpha-tocopherol, although several other forms are also known. It is a preservative because it prevents oxidation in cells, which means it may protect and preserve vitamin A. Although vitamin E has been used extensively in animal research, work done with it on humans has shown that vitamin E does not affect humans and animals the same way. As a result, the role of vitamin E in nutrition has not been scientifically defined. At the same time, widespread claims for vitamin E, for everything from preventing aging and as a "sex vitamin," to curing muscular dystrophy, have been made. Almost none of these properties has been proven in scienific and medical research.

Vitamin E is fat-soluble. It is stored in the fatty, or adipose, tissues and is used along with fat.

Why You Need Vitamin E

The full role of vitamin E in the body is not known. The two properties that have been proven are that vitamin E:

1. Is needed by your body to absorb certain fats.
2. Is necessary to premature and low-birth-weight infants to prevent a form of anemia common in these infants and called hemolytic anemia.

Recommended Daily Allowance

Average adult male	15 IU
Average adult female	12 IU, with needs increasing to 15 IU during pregnancy and while nursing.
Children	Infants need 4-5 IU, with needs increasing to adult RDA in early teens.

Effects of Vitamin E Deficiency

The only known effect is found in premature and low-birth-weight infants, who may develop hemolytic anemia. These infants may be given supplemental vitamin E. One reason for the lack of vitamin E is that the fetus may receive too little because of the faulty transfer of nutrients from the mother to the fetus through the placenta, the organ that connects the fetus to the uterus or womb.

Effects of Excess Vitamin E

Large amounts of vitamin E do not seem to have any effect, either beneficial or harmful, as far as is known.

Sources of Vitamin E

Since no effects of vitamin E deficiency in adults are known, the average balanced diet probably contains enough, if not more than enough, of our daily RDA. Although wheat germ and wheat-germ oil are the richest sources, vitamin E is found in a wide variety of the most common foods. Particularly good sources are vegetable oils (soybean, cottonseed, and corn), nuts, legumes, eggs, liver, leafy vegetables, peanuts, fruits, and margarine.

The abundance of vitamin E in foods may be one reason a deficiency disease can't be found in humans. To reproduce a vitamin E deficiency would mean withholding foods with vitamin E—and that would mean withholding almost all foods.

Cooking Precautions

Vitamin E is relatively stable. It is less apt to be lost in normal preparation and cooking than in processing. Cooking in large amounts of fat is the biggest cause of loss in cooking. As far as processing goes, much vitamin E is known to be lost in milling flour, especially in the bleaching process to make white flour, and in purifying fats to make liquid oils. Rancidity, a natural process, results in oils losing vitamin E as well. Vitamin E can also be destroyed by ultraviolet irradiation and in freezing foods.

History of Vitamin E

Vitamin E was first recognized in the early 1920s and was given its name in 1924. It was then called the "antisterility factor" because it had this effect on rats. No such effect was later found to be true for humans. The Food and Nutrition Board first recognized it as necessary for human nutrition in 1959.

Other Facts

Over the years, more different claims have been made for vitamin E than for any other vitamin. Scientific research has not backed up any of these claims. For one thing, animal research cannot be duplicated in humans, where vitamin E is concerned. Thus, while vitamin E deficiency in rats may cause sterility in males and abnormal termination of pregnancy in females, as well as muscular dystrophy and other diseases, vitamin E has no effect on these conditions and diseases in humans. It has also been called a cure for or preventive of cancer, ulcers, heart disease, and skin disorders and has been used to treat burns. Again, none of these uses have been proven true or even effective. Vitamin E use in such cases can even be harmful, if and when it keeps persons from seeking medical help.

The fact that vitamin E prevents oxidation in cells and acts as a preservative has resulted in some claims that vitamin E prevents aging. This claim seems as groundless as the others.

Nevertheless, vitamin E creams and cosmetics have appeared on the market, based on its supposed antiaging properties. In this respect, you may want to keep in mind what happened after a vitamin E deodorant was introduced in 1973. It later had to be withdrawn from the market because so many people developed rashes, some severe enough for them to have to go to dermatologists for treatment.

Vitamin K

WHAT IS VITAMIN K?

Vitamin K was given its name by its discoverer, who called it K for "koagulation." It is found in foods and is also manufactured in the body by intestinal bacteria.

Vitamin K is oil-soluble. Unlike other oil-soluble vitamins, it is measured in micrograms (μg) instead of international units. Like the other fat-soluble vitamins, it needs bile to be absorbed and is stored in the liver.

Why You Need Vitamin K

Vitamin K is essential for coagulating the blood. The coagulation or clotting is the first step necessary in order for wounds to heal. Four factors in coagulation rely on vitamin K, the most well known of which is prothrombin.

Recommended Daily Allowance

No RDA has been established. Vitamin K is found in a wide variety of foods, with the average daily diet containing about 300 to 500 micrograms of the vitamin. This is more than enough in itself to satisfy daily requirements, without even considering the fact that intestinal bacteria manufacture the vitamin as well.

Effects of Vitamin K Deficiency

Vitamin K deficiency is not seen in the average healthy child and adult. The one exception is in newborn infants, whose intestinal tracts are sterile at birth and cannot manufacture the vitamin. For this reason, they may be given supplemental vitamin K to give them time for the necessary bacteria to develop.

Vitamin K deficiency can develop, however, as the result of a variety of causes. In this case, blood will take longer to clot. Certain antibiotics may be one cause, since they reduce not only disease- or infection-causing bacteria but also other bacteria, including those necessary for making vitamin K. Taking mineral oil can be another cause. It affects the intestines' ability to absorb vitamin K, with a consequent deficiency.

Still another cause is anticoagulant therapy, in which the drugs used act as vitamin K antagonists or antivitamins. This therapy is used to prevent or dissolve blood clots to prevent certain types of strokes and heart attacks.

Some liver disorders can also result in vitamin K deficiency, because the body cannot make adequate use of the vitamin.

Effects of Excess Vitamin K

Very large amounts of vitamin K over a long period of time can be poisonous. The effects, as is the case with too much of other vitamins, can be similar to the vitamin deficiency. It can mean too little prothrombin in the blood, resulting in the inability of the blood to coagulate, certain types of hemorrhages, and kidney disorders.

Sources of Vitamin K

The richest sources are spinach, green cabbage, tomatoes, and pork liver. Good sources are other leafy vegetables (including cauliflower), beef liver, lean meat, and soybean and other vegetable oils.

Cooking Precautions

Vitamin K is stable to heat, light, and exposure to air. It is destroyed by exposure to alkalis, strong acids, and oxidizing agents, as well as ultraviolet light and ionizing rays.

History of Vitamin K

The deficiency was first noticed in the late 1920s in chicks that were fed a diet adequate in all respects except for fat. Their blood clotted normally when alfalfa or hog-liver fat was added. Vitamin K was synthesized in 1939.

Part III
Minerals

Calcium

WHAT IS CALCIUM?

Calcium is an essential mineral or macronutrient. Almost all body calcium is found in bones and teeth. Calcium is what gives the skeleton its rigidity and strength.

Why You Need Calcium

Calcium is needed for many purposes. The most important ones are for the following reasons.

Healthy bones and growth. Bone is constantly being deposited and re-sorbed, which means calcium is needed throughout your life. Your needs are greatest in childhood, especially during adolescence, with its spurt in growth.

The way bone deposition and resorption works is this way: Calcium is car-ried by the blood to the bones, where vitamin D is necessary to activate cal-cium's being deposited in the bone. At the same time that new bone is being deposited, old bone is being resorbed into the bloodstream. In children, more bone is deposited than is resorbed, thus accounting for growth. Once maximum growth is reached, the deposition and resorption balance out until old age, when bone resorption is greater than bone deposition.

The bones also store calcium for other uses. If you don't get enough calcium daily, the body relies on these stores, getting what it needs by resorbing or mobilizing the calcium from the bones. During childhood, if the child does not get enough calcium or vitamin D, the resorption results in rickets. (See vitamin D.) In old age, the changes resulting from greater resorption than deposition are called osteoporosis. In both rickets and osteoporosis, the lack of calcium means that bones become fragile and break easily. Such resorption, however, can happen at any age if calcium is lacking.

Healthy teeth. Calcium is especially important to the fetus before birth and through childhood and adolescence when both baby teeth and second teeth are erupting and growing. Once teeth have grown, the calcium in them is relatively stable with very little deposition and resorption. The lack of calcium in youth and improper formation of teeth, however, may lead to cavities in later life.

Muscle contraction and expansion. When muscles contract or expand, cal-cium is drawn into them. When muscles relax, the calcium is withdrawn by the surrounding cells. Calcium, therefore, is essential to the functioning of the heart and its regular expansion and contraction.

Clotting of the blood. Calcium is needed by the plasma, the liquid in which the red and white blood cells are suspended, for the blood to clot. In case of injury, the calcium is mobilized to stimulate the red blood cells in a series of chain reactions that produce a substance called fibrin. The actual clot, then, is composed of fibrin.

Recommended Daily Allowance
Average adult male	800 mg
Average adult female	800 mg, with needs increasing to 1,200 mg during pregnancy and while nursing.
Children	Infants' needs increase from 360 mg to 800 mg during childhood and to 1,200 mg during adolescence. After age 18, the adult RDA of 800 mg suffices.

Effects of Calcium Deficiency
Low blood calcium decreases the blood's ability to clot and may cause muscular twitching, spasms, and convulsions. In infancy and childhood, severe calcium deficiency results in rickets. In adults, lack of calcium may be a cause of osteoporosis.

Effects of Excess Calcium
None.

Sources of Calcium
The best sources are milk and yogurt, cream, cheese, egg yolks, beans, cauliflower, chard, kale, molasses, and rhubarb. Good sources are beets, carrots, leafy vegetables (cabbage, kohlrabi, lettuce, spinach, watercress), celery, parsnips, rutabagas, turnips, almonds, and walnuts, bran, oatmeal, chocolate, dates, figs, lemons, oranges, pineapples, raspberries, shellfish, and oysters.

Cooking Precautions
Cooking causes slight losses of calcium in vegetables, since the mineral tends to wash out in cooking water.

Other Facts
Calcium often needs phosphorus in order to form the compounds that can be used by your body. Calcium in combination with phosphorus is especially important for bone growth and maintenance and for teeth.

Chlorine

WHAT IS CHLORINE?

Chlorine is an essential mineral or macronutrient. It is found in the body in compounds called chlorides, combinations of chlorine with other elements. Sodium chloride (salt) is the most common compound.

Why You Need Chlorine

Chlorides help regulate metabolism and the flow of liquids between cells (osmosis). Osmosis is essential to the maintenance of the functions of your body. Chlorine in the form of hydrochloric acid is important to digestion.

Recommended Daily Allowance

There is no RDA. The average diet contains the 3 to 9 grams considered necessary.

Effects of Chlorine Deficiency

None. The only time that your body may not have enough chlorine is after vomiting. This chlorine is restored through foods.

Effects of Excess Chlorine

Excess chlorine is excreted in the urine and in perspiration. Perspiration is basically sodium chloride (salt).

Sources of Chlorine

The only special source is table salt. Almost every kind of food contains salt as well.

Cooking Precautions

None.

Other Facts

Chlorine has germicidal properties, which is why it is used—much diluted—to treat water supplies to make them safe to drink. It is also a bleach. In this respect, strong concentrations of chlorine are poisonous and can burn the mucous membranes and respiratory passages. For these reasons, products and preparations containing chlorine (such as household bleaches) should be used carefully and stored where children can't reach them.

Chromium

WHAT IS CHROMIUM?

Chromium is an essential trace element or micronutrient.

Why You Need Chromium

Chromium plays a role in the metabolism of glucose, the form of carbohydrates made by the body after digestion and used by the body as fuel or energy. It may also have a role in how the body uses the hormone, insulin.

Other Facts

Too little is known about chromium and its role in the body for any recommended daily allowance to be established.

It is found in yeast, some animal products (excluding fish), and whole grains.

Cobalt

WHAT IS COBALT?

Cobalt is an essential trace element or micronutrient.

Other Facts

Cobalt is a component of vitamin B_{12}. As a result it is necessary in the production of red blood cells and the prevention of certain kinds of anemia. It is found in the same foods that contain vitamin B_{12}.

Copper

WHAT IS COPPER?

Copper is an essential trace element or micronutrient.

Why You Need Copper

Copper is essential, along with iron, to the making of the blood's hemoglobin. Certain enzymes necessary to metabolism also contain copper.

Recommended Daily Allowance

The RDA has been estimated to be

Average adult male   2.0 mg
Average adult female   2.0 mg
Children   Infants need from 0.05-0.1 mg, with requirements increasing to adult RDA in adolescence.

Effects of Copper Deficiency

Because of its importance to hemoglobin, lack of copper may result in anemia. In this respect it may affect the body's ability to use iron. Respiration and growth are affected by lack of copper, too.

Effects of Excess Copper

Unknown.

Sources of Copper

Rich sources of copper include crustaceans and shellfish (especially oysters), organ meats (liver, kidney, and brains), dried legumes and nuts, raisins, and cocoa. Leafy green vegetables are a good source of copper, depending on the copper in the soil where they are grown. This last resource, therefore, is unreliable. Also, some drinking waters contain copper.

Fluorine

WHAT IS FLUORINE?

Fluorine is an essential trace element or micronutrient. It is found naturally in soil along with calcium.

Why You Need Fluorine

Fluorine is found in bones and teeth, especially in dental enamel. Since fluorine prevents the formation of cavities, it is related to healthy teeth.

Recommended Daily Allowance

Unknown.

Effects of Flourine Deficiency

Fluorine deficiency is related to increased susceptibility to dental cavities, particularly in children.

In adults, recent research has indicated that there may be a relationship between fluorine deficiency and osteoporosis in older women and between fluorine deficiency and atherosclerosis or hardening of the arteries in men. In areas where drinking water is rich in fluorine, these diseases seem to be less in number.

Effects of Excess Fluorine

Certain areas, such as the Panhandle area in Texas, have a very high natural amount of fluorine in the water. This high concentration—which is much higher than the amount added to water in other areas to prevent cavities—has been linked to the formation of mottled dental enamel in the children who live there.

Sources of Fluorine

Fluoridated water is the best source, since amounts of fluorine in foods depend on the fluorine in the soil in which they are grown.

Iodine

WHAT IS IODINE?

Iodine is a trace element or micronutrient. Despite the fact that your body requires less iodine than it does of essential minerals, iodine is vital to the health and well-being of your body.

Why You Need Iodine

Iodine is vital in preventing goiter, an enlargement of the thyroid gland in the neck. It is both a part of the gland and is used by the gland in making certain hormones that regulate metabolism and the release of body energy. If not enough iodine is available, another gland—the pituitary—makes a hormone that activates the thyroid gland to make more of its hormones. This stimulation causes the thyroid gland to grow larger, resulting in the swelling in the neck, which is typical of goiter.

Recommended Daily Allowance

Average adult male 130μg

Average adult female 100μg, with needs increasing to 125μg during pregnancy and to 150μg while nursing.

Children   Infants need 35μg, with requirements increasing to 150μg for boys, and 115μg for girls at age 11 before decreasing to adult RDA at about age 20.

Effects of Iodine Deficiency

Goiter is the result of iodine deficiency. In children, however, lack of enough iodine can lead to mental and physical retardation.

If the thyroid gland produces too little of its hormones, the result is hypothyroidism, which is marked by sluggish metabolism. The person may be listless, with a tendency toward obesity and slowed body activity.

Effects of Excess Iodine

Excess iodine in itself is not a problem, but an overactive thyroid gland can result in the production of too many of the gland's hormones (hyperthyroidism). In hyperthyroidism, a person is nervous and irritable, with a tendency to lose weight despite an increased appetite.

Sources of Iodine

The amount of iodine in foods varies greatly. For example, the amount of iodine in plants depends on the amount of iodine in the soil. In turn, the amount of iodine in meats and dairy products depends on the amount of iodine in the animal's feed.

Iodine is also found in drinking water, and that amount varies from one locality to another. For these reasons, a major source of iodine is iodized table salt.

Cooking Precautions

Because the amount of iodine varies so greatly, iodized table salt should be used in preparing and cooking foods.

Other Facts

Iodine was one of the first trace elements found to be vital to the body's nutrition. Since 1895 it has been used to treat goiter.

Goiter seems to run in patterns, depending on and corresponding to the iodine content of soil, water, and foods. Japan, for example, has the lowest proportion of goiter of any other area because of its dependence on seafoods and especially seaweed. Yet in other areas of the world goiter is an endemic condition due to diet and other factors.

In the United States, the use of iodized salt has drastically reduced endemic goiter. Also, because foods are grown in so many places and shipped around the country, there is less distinction of goiter from one area to another. One point to keep in mind is that commercially prepared foods, from canned foods to frozen meals, which contain salt, rarely use iodized salt.

Iron

WHAT IS IRON?

Iron is a trace element or micronutrient. The body's needs for iron, however, greatly outweigh the amount of iron found in the body.

Why You Need Iron

You need iron to make hemoglobin, the red cells of the blood. Although it also has a role in keeping certain tissues healthy, the majority of iron is needed by and used in the blood. It is absorbed from food in the small intestine and is carried by the blood to the bone marrow where it is used to make the red blood cells' hemoglobin. Red blood cells live for about 120 days, after which time their iron is reused to make new cells. The formation of hemoglobin requires copper. Vitamins B_{12}, C, and E also have a function in maintaining hemoglobin.

Recommended Daily Allowance

Average adult male	10 mg
Average adult female	18 mg, with additional iron required during pregnancy and while nursing. Women need more iron because 0.5-1.0 mg of iron are lost *every day* during menstruation. After menopause (when the childbearing years are over), a woman's needs are the same as a man's.
Children	Infants require 10 mg, with their needs increasing to 15 mg through 3 years and to 18 mg during adolescence. By 18 or 19, boys' needs are the same as the average adult male's, with girls' needs remaining at 18 mg, the same as the average adult female's.

Effects of Iron Deficiency

A lack of iron leads to anemia. The symptoms are a lowered vitality and paleness. In children, an iron deficiency can lead to retarded development.

Effects of Excess Iron

The problem is to get enough iron. The body is remarkably efficient in using iron, with iron being stored in the liver, spleen, and mucous membranes of the intestines. Any excess iron is disposed of by the intestines in the feces.

Sources of Iron

Calves or lambs liver is the richest source of iron, followed by beef and chicken liver. Other excellent food sources are meat, fish, poultry, green leafy vegetables, potatoes, legumes, egg yolks, dried fruits, and enriched breads and cereals. Molasses and raisins are excellent sources, too, but are probably not used regularly enough and in sufficient quantities to be reliable sources.

The richest sources of iron, incidentally, are those foods with the richest color. Spinach, for example, has more iron than iceberg lettuce; egg yolks, more than egg whites; molasses, more than refined white sugar; and whole wheat bread, more than white bread (depending on the latter's enrichment).

Milk is *not* a good source of iron.

Cooking Precautions

Using iron cookware will increase the iron content of foods because a certain amount of iron is absorbed by the foods from utensils.

Other Facts

The average adult male who eats a balanced diet should get his RDA of iron from foods. Children, and women during their child-bearing years, may require supplementary iron, since they may not get enough iron even if they eat additional iron-rich foods.

Magnesium

WHAT IS MAGNESIUM?

Magnesium is an essential mineral or macronutrient. It is the essential mineral found in the smallest quantity in the body. About half or slightly more than half is found in the bones, along with calcium and phosphorus. The rest is found in other body cells, mainly in the muscles and red blood cells.

Why You Need Magnesium

Magnesium mobilizes the enzymes used in the metabolism of fats, carbohydrates, and especially protein. It helps regulate your body temperature and is involved in muscular contraction.

Recommended Daily Allowance

Average adult male	350 mg
Average adult female	300 mg with needs increasing to 450 mg during pregnancy and while nursing.
Children	Infants require 60 mg, with needs increasing to adult RDA between the ages of 11 and 14. The exception is boys between the ages of 15 and 18, their period of greatest growth, who need 400 mg.

Effects of Magnesium Deficiency

Magnesium deficiency is similar to calcium deficiency. The symptoms are muscular spasms that can result in convulsions, weakness, and depression. Because magnesium helps regulate muscular contractions, its deficiency may also result in an irregular heart beat.

Effects of Excess Magnesium

The effects of excess magnesium require further research. One observation is that high magnesium levels and intake is, in some way, related to low calcium levels in soft tissues such as blood vessels and a lower incidence of heart disease. At this point, however, this relationship is not understood or defined by those in the field.

Sources of Magnesium

The average diet contains more than adequate levels of magnesium. Increased needs, such as in adolescent boys, and in pregnant women, are normally met by their increased need and consumption of calories.

Magnesium is found in a wide variety of foods, including meats, milk, seafood, green vegetables, cereal grains, nuts, legumes, and cocoa.

Cooking Precautions

None.

Other Facts

Certain diseases and disorders decrease the body's ability to absorb and make use of magnesium. These include diabetes, chronic alcoholism, some kidney diseases, disorders of the parathyroid gland, and disorders in which the ability of the body to absorb magnesium is genetically impaired.

Magnesium in the bones is far more stable than calcium and is not readily transferred between bones and tissues.

Manganese

WHAT IS MANGANESE?

Manganese is an essential trace element or micronutrient.

Why You Need Manganese

Manganese is required for bone growth and is a component of many enzymes.

Recommended Daily Allowance
Average adult   2–3 mg
Children   Not established

Effects of Manganese Deficiency
None, as far as is known.

Effects of Excess Manganese
None, as far as is known.

Sources of Manganese
Nuts, whole grains, legumes, tea, cloves, bananas, blueberries, beets, and chocolate are among the best sources. The amount of manganese in fruits and vegetables may be affected by the manganese in the soil in which they are grown.

Meat, fish, and dairy products contain little manganese.

Molybdenum

WHAT IS MOLYBDENUM?

Molybdenum is an essential trace element or micronutrient.

Why You Need Molybdenum

Molybdenum is a component of certain enzymes essential for metabolism.

Other Facts

Too little is known about this element for a recommended daily allowance to be established. In addition, there is no known deficiency disease.

Good sources are beef kidney, legumes, and some cereals.

Phosphorus

WHAT IS PHOSPHORUS?

Phosphorus is an essential mineral or macronutrient, second only to calcium in the amount found in the body. It is usually found in bones and teeth in combination with calcium.

Why You Need Phosphorus

Phosphorus, like calcium, is essential to the formation, growth, and maintenance of healthy bones and teeth. It is also required by the muscles and, to a lesser extent, by nerve tissues. Also, phosphorus is necessary to the body's use of fats and fatty acids. Phosphorus is absorbed and metabolized with the help of vitamin D.

Recommended Daily Allowance

Average adult male   800 mg

Average adult female   800 mg, with needs increasing to 1,200 mg during pregnancy and while nursing.

Children: Infants' needs increase from 240 mg to a high of 1,200 mg during the high-growth years between 11 and 18, after which needs decrease to adult RDA.

Effects of Phosphorus Deficiency

Phosphorus deficiency in children results in retarded growth, faulty formation of bones and teeth, and rickets—the same as with calcium and vitamin D deficiencies. Low levels of phosphorus at any age can mean a loss of weight and feelings of weakness.

A person with a phosphorus deficiency may have a perverted appetite—that is, a desire for substances containing phosphorus that are not foods. A craving for chalk, clay, talc, or such substances is often noticed among people whose diets are deficient in this essential mineral.

Effects of Excess Phosphorus
The phosphorus that the body cannot use is excreted in the urine.

Sources of Phosphorus
Proteins are the finest sources of phosphorus. The best sources are liver, milk, eggs, lentils, beans, barley, bran, oatmeal, whole wheat and rye products, almonds, walnuts, peanuts, peas, cocoa, and chocolate. Good sources are beef, chicken, fish, clams, cream; such vegetables as asparagus, cauliflower, cabbage, carrots, celery, chard, corn, cucumbers, egg plant, and green beans; and such fruits as figs, prunes, pineapple, pumpkin, and raisins.

Cooking Precautions
Some phosphorus may be lost in cooking water.

Other Facts
Phosphorus in itself is poisonous, which is why some rat and roach poisons contain it. For this reason, these poisons should be kept in a safe place, especially where children can't find or easily reach them. Although modern safety matches contain no phosphorus, phosphorus poisoning from matches used to be common among children.

Potassium

WHAT IS POTASSIUM?

Potassium is an essential mineral or macronutrient. Although it is third to calcium and phosphorus, it is found in the body in much smaller quantities than these other two essential minerals; but it is just as essential to the body's functions.

Why You Need Potassium

Potassium is found primarily in the body's fluids. It is essential for the maintenance of a proper fluid balance and for the transferrence of nutrients between and among cells to meet the body's nutrition requirements. Potassium, along with calcium and magnesium, is needed for contraction of muscles. It is also required by the nervous system.

Recommended Daily Allowance

No RDA has been established because potassium is found in so many foods that the average diet contains more potassium than the body needs.

Effects of Potassium Deficiency

The average person, child or adult, is not likely to develop a potassium deficiency. Certain medications, however, do affect the body's use of potassium. These include diuretics, such as those used to lower high blood pressure or hypertension. Persons taking such medications should take care to eat potassium-rich foods.

Vomiting and diarrhea may also cause a temporary potassium deficiency because of the body's inability to make use of foods. Foods, including fruit juices, are the major way to restore the potassium balance.

Potassium is a major component of the liquid used in the intravenous feeding of seriously ill patients who are unable to eat regular foods. It is essential.to help these persons maintain as normal a fluid balance as possible.

Deficiency symptoms include dizziness, thirst, mental confusion, and weakness of the muscles.

Effects of Excess Potassium
Excess potassium is excreted.

Sources of Potassium
The best sources are fresh vegetables, fresh and dried fruit, cereals, dried peas and beans, nuts, molasses, cocoa, fresh fish, and fresh poultry. Almonds, dried apricots, bananas, avocados, and Brazil nuts are exceptionally good sources.

Selenium

WHAT IS SELENIUM

Selenium is an essential trace element or micronutrient.

Other Facts

Selenium has been identified as having a role in animal nutrition, especially in preventing the degeneration of the liver and muscles. In animals, it may also be related to the effectiveness of vitamin E. The relationship of these roles to human nutrition hasn't been proven.

Selenium in foods depends on the amount in the soil in which they are grown.

Sodium

WHAT IS SODIUM?

Sodium is an essential mineral or macronutrient. It is found in the body's fluids and tissues, most commonly in the form of salt (sodium chloride).

Why You Need Sodium

Sodium helps preserve the body's fluid balance by preventing an excessive loss of water that could lead to dehydration. It also helps maintain a normal heartbeat by preserving the proper relationship between calcium and potassium in the heart's muscles. In addition, it is necessary to the nervous system and the transmitting of nerve impulses.

Recommended Daily Allowance

No RDA has been established because salt is so plentiful in almost all foods and more is usually added to flavor food.

Effects of Sodium Deficiency

The abundance of salt in the diet makes sodium deficiency impossible under normal circumstances. The time when a salt deficiency becomes a distinct possibility is through excessive sweating, when salt is excreted along with water. The reason may be a fever or high summer temperatures. In either case, the person should drink plenty of liquids to restore the body fluids. In the summer, when sweating is apt to continue for an extended period of time, taking salt tablets with a large amount of water may be necessary.

Effects of Excess Sodium

Liberal salting of foods and a diet based on salty foods have been linked to high blood pressure or hypertension. If blood pressure gets high enough, salt can literally be a killer because high blood pressure is a primary cause of stroke and heart disease. Persons with high blood pressure, therefore, are wise to reduce their use of salt and to stay away from excessively salty foods. They cannot avoid salt altogether, because all foods contain salt.

Sources of Sodium

The wide availability of salt can be shown by the fact that both whole and skimmed milk contain 15 milligrams of salt in each 100 grams. If you wish to avoid salt as much as possible, you should avoid the foods with the highest salt content, such as bacon and especially Canadian bacon, corn flakes, Parmesan and Cheddar cheese, crab meat, sardines, soda crackers, salted butter and margarine, olives and especially green olives, dill pickles, potato chips, pretzels, French and Italian salad dressings, and catsup.

Cooking Precautions

If you're on a low-salt or salt-free diet, do not use salt in the cooking water. It may add flavor but it increases your sodium intake, even though you may not add more salt at the table. Lemon juice and spices can be substituted to add flavor.

Other Facts

If you do and can use salt, use iodized salt to supply the iodine your body needs as well as sodium.

If you're on a reducing diet, remember that a good portion of weight is due to water. One reason you may appear to lose weight quickly at first is that certain foods taken in large quantities (as often happens on diets) act as diuretics, substances that withdraw water from the tissues. Some of these diets can be dangerous, since they may upset the normal fluid balance and can cause symptoms of dehydration. Even though a weight loss may be desirable from a point of view of health (overweight contributes to a variety of diseases, including high blood pressure), no diet should be undertaken without a physician's advice and supervision.

If you're on a salt-free diet, read labels on commercially prepared foods. These often contain added salt. In this respect, many commercial baby foods contain salt, too. The reason is less because of nutritional value and children's tastes than because parents taste the foods. This salt is not essential, according to nutritionists and medical authorities, and may even be harmful in giving infants an acquired taste for salt early in life, thus contributing to high blood pressure in later life.

Sulfur

WHAT IS SULFUR?

Sulfur is an essential mineral or macronutrient. It is a component of the protein found in all cells and is in both human cells and food proteins.

Why You Need Sulfur

You need sulfur to make keratin, a tough protein essential to hair and nails. Sulfur is also necessary to the chemical makeup of various other compounds used by the body, such as thiamine and biotin in the vitamin family; the hormone, insulin; and others.

Recommended Daily Allowance

No RDA has been established, but since sulfur is found in most protein you get more than enough sulfur if you eat a sufficient amount of protein.

Effects of Sulfur Deficiency

Lack of sulfur can result in dermatitis and improper growth of hair and nails. Severe deficiency of certain sulfur compounds can mean restricted growth because of its relationship to protein.

Effects of Excess Sulfur

None, as far as is known.

Sources of Sulfur

All protein foods, both animal and vegetables.

Cooking Precautions

None.

Other Facts

Certain sulfur compounds used by industry can be poisonous. Care should be taken in handling or working with sulfur dioxide and sulfuric acid, among others.

Zinc

WHAT IS ZINC?

Zinc is an essential trace element or micronutrient. It is found in animal and plant tissues in amounts second only to iron among the trace elements.

Why You Need Zinc

Zinc is a component of hair, skin, eyes, and nails, and of the testes in men. It is also involved with metabolism. In addition, insulin—the hormone that regulates the metabolism and maintenance of the proper level of blood sugar, thus preventing diabetes—contains zinc.

Recommended Daily Allowance

The RDA for zinc was established for the first time by the Food and Nutrition Board in 1974. It is:

Average adult male	15 mg
Average adult female	15 mg, with needs increasing to 20 mg during pregnancy and to 25 mg while nursing.
Children	Infants' needs start at 3 mg, increasing to 10 mg at 1 year of age and to 15 mg at age 11.

Effects of Zinc Deficiency

Marginal zinc deficiency results in a poor sense of taste, a poor appetite, slow healing of wounds, and less than normal growth. More severe deficiency can result in dwarfism, certain kinds of anemia, and defective secretion of both male and female sex glands.

Effects of Excess Zinc

None, as far as is known.

Sources of Zinc

The best sources are beef, Cheddar cheese, cocoa, seafoods (especially raw oysters and crab meat), egg yolks, poultry hearts and gizzards, lamb, liver, oatmeal and oat products, peanuts, peas, popcorn, pork, veal, wheat germ, and whole wheat products.

Your body is better able to absorb zinc from animal foods than from legumes and grains. Vegetarians, therefore, run a greater risk of zinc deficiency than do meat and fish eaters.

Cooking Precautions

Some zinc is lost in cooking vegetables and legumes in water.

Other Facts

Certain medications make use of zinc for its antiseptic and astringent properties.

Alcohol affects the ability of the body to use zinc. As a result, chronic alcoholism can result in zinc deficiency.

Other Trace Elements

Many other elements have been found in tissues of plants and animals, including humans. What roles these elements play and how much may be essential remains to be learned. In the meantime, certain facts are known about some of these trace elements:

Cadmium. Cadmium is a trace element that is found in water, especially soft water. Some research has linked it to hypertension and heart disease and stroke. In areas where water is soft, with high levels of cadmium, the rate of hypertension and heart disease has been found to be higher than in areas where water is hard and low in cadmium.

Lead. Lead is a trace element that can be dangerous in large amounts. Although lead is present in the air and in food and water, the major danger of lead poisoning is with children and occurs in the home. Lead has been used in wall paints, woodwork, and toys and in glazes for ceramics. It is also used with silver to make pewter. Lead poisoning in children who chewed or ate the flakes of paint led to its being banned for use in paints. At the same time, many old houses may still contain undercoats of lead paints that children can get at and ingest into their systems. Lead poisoning can lead to mental retardation and permanent neurological damage.

Mercury. Mercury that has been dumped into the water as industrial wastes can lead to mercury poisoning. Even though the water is not drunk, fish can consume the mercury, with the result that humans who eat the fish may be poisoned. For this reason, mercury levels in water and fish are monitored, with high mercury levels leading to the condemning of fishing grounds.

Other trace elements may be beneficial. Lithium, for example, has been found to be effective in treating manic depression.

Glossary

Alkali A substance that combines with an acid and water to form a salt. Baking soda is an alkali that combines with constituents of food to destroy vitamin C and other vitamins.

Amino Acid The end product of protein metabolism. Proteins are composed of many amino acids linked together.

Antagonist A substance that acts in such a way as to destroy or neutralize a vitamin to make it unable to do its work. Avidin in raw egg white and certain antibiotics are vitamin antagonists. Some vitamin antagonists may be medically useful. See vitamin K.

Antivitamin See *vitamin antagonist*.

Calorie The amount of food necessary to produce a unit of heat, also called a calorie. The calories eaten should be equal to the energy expended. If more calories, in this ratio, are eaten, we gain weight. If less are eaten, we lose weight, provided the energy expenditure is the same.

Carbohydrate A major food group that includes sugars, starches, and celluloses.

Coenzyme A substance that activates an enzyme. Vitamins may be coenzymes of specific enzymes.

Collagen The "cement" or "glue" that holds cells and tissues together. It is also necessary to the healing of wounds and bones. Vitamin C is essential to the formation of collagen.

DNA Deoxyribonucleic acid, which with RNA forms the chemical basis of heredity and carries the cells' genetic information.

Enzyme A chemical substance formed in the body and found especially in digestive juices. Enzymes are necessary to break down the food we eat into simple products the body can use. Enzymes, for example, break protein down into amino acids.

Essential Mineral A mineral, such as calcium, that is needed by and used in the body in large quantities. The amount is relative, however, to the minute quantities required of trace elements.

Fat An organic compound insoluble in water. Fats, along with proteins and carbohydrates, are a major source of the body's fuel.

Fat-Soluble Substances that can be dissolved in fats. Certain vitamins (A, D, E, and K) are soluble only in fats and, thus, can be stored in the body.

Fatty Acid An end product of fat metabolism.

Glucose An end product of carbohydrate metabolism. Glucose is a major source of the body's energy.

Glycerol An end product of fat metabolism.

Gram A unit of measurement in the metric system: 1 ounce = 28.3 grams.

Hormone A substance that stimulates the functioning of the body. Hormones are essential for growth, sexual activity, and a variety of other purposes. Insulin, a hormone produced by the pancreas, is essential for the metabolism and maintenance of blood sugar. Certain vitamins act as prohormones, which means their presence is necessary for the organ, gland, or some other part of the body to produce the hormone.

International Unit (IU) A measurement, roughly equivalent to a milligram, used to measure the biologic activity of fat-soluble vitamins.

Lactovegetarian A vegetarian diet that includes milk and dairy products (lacto) as well as fruits and vegetables.

Macronutrient Another name for an essential mineral. *Macro* means "large." Thus, a macronutrient is a mineral required in large amounts.

Megavitamin A vitamin taken in large amounts. The amounts are much higher than those given under the recommended daily allowances.

Metabolism The sum of the body's processes in breaking down the food eaten into substances the body can use and the use the body makes of those substances.

Microgram A unit of measurement in the metric system: 1 gram = 1,000,000 micrograms.

Micronutrient Another name for a trace element. *Micro means* "small." Thus, a micronutrient is a mineral required in small, often minute or trace, quantities.

Microgram A unit of measurement in the metric system: 1 gram = 1,000,000 micrograms.

Mineral An element or substance that is unique and basic in that it cannot be broken down into any simpler substance. Minerals consist of essential minerals and trace elements. Although found in foods and the human body, they are not of organic (animal or plant) origin, but are found in soil and water.

Organic A carbon compound of animal or plant origin. Vitamins are organic, or carbon, compounds that can be synthesized once the chemical structure is known, using their elements. As the word is used in a natural- or health-food sense, it means a food grown without the use of chemical fertilizers and pesticides. The preferred term is "organically grown."

Osmosis The passage of liquids through membranes. The body's fluid balance depends on osmosis of fluids containing certain minerals, such as sodium, chlorine, and potassium.

Ovolactovegetarian A vegetarian (fruit and vegetable) diet that includes milk and dairy products (lacto) and eggs (ovo).

Precursor A substance that comes before another substance. Certain substances are precursors of vitamins and, thus, are provitamins. Some vitamins may be precursors of hormones and, thus, are prohormones.

Preformed A vitamin that is complete in the form in which it is found in foods. Vitamin A, for example, is preformed only in animal products. The form found in vegetables is carotene, which is a vitamin A precursor, or provitamin, that must be converted into vitamin A during the digestive process.

Prohormone See *precursor.*

Protein The food group consisting of animal products and certain kinds of vegetables, such as legumes.

Provitamin See *precursor*

RDA Recommended Daily Allowance. The RDA or amount of vitamins and minerals necessary to the health and maintenance of the body is established by the Food and Nutrition Board of the National Research Council/National Academy of Science.

Retinol Equivalent (RE) A unit of measurement of the biologic activity of retinol, the active compound of vitamin A.

RNA See *DNA*

Trace Elements Minerals required by the body in a lesser amount than essential minerals. See *micronutrient.*

Vegans A vegetarian diet in which only fruits and vegetables are consumed. No animal products are eaten.

Vitamin Organic compounds found in foods. They don't add to the weight, change the taste, or contribute calories.

Water-Soluble A substance soluble in water and not in fat. Vitamins C and B are water-soluble, with the excess generally excreted in urine or through perspiration.